Surviving Cancer

Kay D. Quain

with Jack Coyle

Sheed & Ward

Sheed & Ward™ is a service of National Catholic Reporter Publishing
Company, Inc.

Library of Congress Catalog Card Number: 88-62065

ISBN: 1-55612-156-3

Published by: Sheed & Ward
                115 E. Armour Blvd. P.O. Box 419492
                Kansas City, MO 64141

To order, call: (800) 333-7373

Contents

October 14, 1981

The leaf pranced and danced, falling, until it came to rest at my feet. So beautiful. Why must it wither and die? A paradox. I am standing in the autumn bluster on the path outside my doctor's office.

Autumn is nature's paradox. There is awesome beauty in her dance and yet, it is a dance of dying.

I have cancer. But I'll fight this thought of death—just like the chemotherapy, just injected, will help me fight this rebellion, this mutiny inside my body.

It is truly a beautiful autumn day. I am aggressively alive, and there is pungent promise in the air. And I know there will be a tomorrow.

Preface

My family is my strength. I have been their's and now there exists a dynamic give and take of this sustenance. They have endured so very much in these past twenty months. First there was diagnosis and then surgery. It comes at you brutal and fast if you let it. Now I must tell them more upsetting news: more surgery. I am too tired now to feel much anxiety. I cannot manage the theatrics needed to tell them like I want to, so I wait.

"You have cancer": might be the ultimate assault upon a person. It comes at you relentless, like an ocean wave and turns and spins you and knocks you among the rocks and ancient shells before it beaches you. Mine was much metastasized. A rebellion long in process, not found out until the mutineers were rallying at the palace gate.

One does not wish to be a statistic on a page. I am part of a living universe. I am an integral star, shining, defiant and bright. I will not, I do not wish to be dimmed and darkened by some part of me gone awry.

I am but one of thousands, however, stricken with cancer this year. It is 1980 and I am not a mere statistic and I do not want to die.

Introduction

I shall confess to you my love of a challenge. Rather than love, call it a certain tenacity, an approach toward life that seeks 'right' or 'justice', or maybe just survival. Toward any adversity we have a choice. We can either be passive and allow this world to have her way with us, or we can rebel and apply whatever force within us to a particular fray.

If this intruder and I are to war for the months and years ahead, I must arm my commitment with a powerful arsenal.

Cancer challenges me to become a partner with the medical profession. We each have roles to play here. They plot the course of a focused medical assault. I assume responsibility for all else aimed at making me well.

I must embrace surgery, stringent chemotherapy, endless testing. This is medicine and it is my ally. I must congeal my own resources. My spirit and my mind must focus toward healing my body.

I am at war with 'THE BIG C.' I mean to win and will, therefore, summon the forces of my faith, attitudinal therapy, meditation and imagery to fight this fight. My strategy, as this war weakens my physical reserve, is to bolster myself with faith in who and what I am and trust in my healing medical partners.

My purpose in writing is simple. I want to help cancer patients and their families. Cancer affects everyone in a family and so I invite all of you along with me on my intense and personal war, and that of my family, against this disease. We say that love knows no bounds. It is true. Friends of a cancer patient provide a needed and very special part of a total resource: human warmth. I ask that you realize this. If you are a patient, seek this. If you are a friend or part of family, give it with all your heart. It is one single thing this world has to offer which, even by itself, offers boundless reason and resource to live.

There is no scale to measure what helped me most in my battle. I believe it was a combination, a focus of many resources that allowed me to hold on through this wrenching time. I won. My family and my doctors won too. There are years ahead.

1.
The Diagnosis

Life

God asks no man whether he will accept Life.
That is not the choice. You must take it.
The only choice is how?

Henry Ward Beecher

Winter 1980

My body is overly warm in spite of the cold. It is a blustery Thursday
in February. I drive hurriedly home from the doctor through crunching
snow with dull pain in my left lower abdomen. The pain is coming center
stage; coming to the center of my world. Damn it, Why could it not have
been insignificant!

The examination of my pelvis worries my doctor. And he's sent me off
to see a surgeon in the emergency room immediately. He says I'll probably
be admitted.

I get home, put some essentials into an overnight bag and tell my family. We hurry out.

1

I am admitted following the surgeon's examination. My pain is tolerable, even familiar. I had had two previous operations in exactly the same place years ago. A strangulated hernia. I think perhaps it needs repair again, nothing more than that.

Testing takes two days. "We have detected a mass in your left lower pelvic region and a tumor is evident in the right." The surgeon is crisp and confident. "Surgery is scheduled for Monday," he says.

Exploratory surgery will determine if both a hernia and diverticulitis are present in my left side, along the with the tumor on the right. My speculation runs the gamut and behind it all is a clammy glimmer that it could be cancer.

I analyze my situation and pray hard for a favorable outcome. Sleep is sporadic but I am confident that I have outguessed the surgeon. Ever the optimist. When I wake from surgery I know the key question to ask. "Did they remove my uterus?" A fibroid tumor had been detected in my uterus two years ago. I am told that the uterus is also oversized. It is logical then to remove it. If they answer yes to my question then, in all probability, I would get favorable news post-surgery.

Do I or do I not have cancer? Now I will secretly know the answer to that question before someone else must take on the assignment of telling me. I remain uncertain how I will deal with negative news.

There is a blur of white and surgical green. I fight through the anesthesia in glimpses. "Did they remove my uterus," I ask. I could not distinguish the face but the voice was feminine, gentle and held a sympathetic edge. "No dear," she said. "Try and sleep now. The doctor will talk with you later."

I have cancer. The knowledge cut through and merged with the dwindling effect of the drugs. I knew there was a possibility but I really did not expect this result, this unofficial tally. I try and ready myself for the pending disclosure and wonder how it will be handled.

I sleep through the rest of that Monday through the afternoon and the night.

It is Tuesday morning and I am back in my room. Confident of my ability to handle the news yet defensive, wondering from where it will come. I plan to meet this with a positive comment but wonder if I can carry it off.

The passing hours irritate me. I want to hear the words. I want to get this over with. My confidence wavers and I stifle an urge to pose the question, straight away to the next nurse I see. "DO I have cancer, or do you even know?" No. I will not do this. I'll play by medical rules and wait for the 'right' person.

Throughout this endless day nurses come and go and avoid my eyes. Everyone is bustling about performing their chores and making inconsequential banter. I feel like the eye of a storm and want desperately for someone to reach out to me. A tension seems to build around me. All the familiar faces now smile from far away. No one will make contact.

I know and they do not know that I know. This thought amuses me. Not for long.

Suddenly I understand that it will be my family who will break this devastating news to me. Where are they? When is someone going to tell me? My daughter calls. She asks how I am doing and I lie that I am doing fine. I startle at the thought that she has been chosen to tell me. Not so.

Residents arrive to inspect the incision, remove bandages and tubes. They completely avoid looking into my eyes. My every question is met with the same reply: "How does the incision look?" "Fine." "How am I doing?" "Fine." Quickly they remove themselves from the hot seat. "The surgeon will be here to talk with you."

I want to scream. "Why doesn't someone tell me so that you all know that I know? I am determined to be capable of handling this news!" Let's get on with Life!

The hours following this surgery are the loneliest time of my life.

The choreography of this disclosure begins at mid-afternoon. My roommate tells me she is leaving the room. As the door closes to her leaving, my husband Bill appears. He is drained and has been crying and with the first words from his lips he weeps openly again. He, my husband and friend of 29 years, says these words: "I must tell you that you have cancer." Tears stream down his face and he clutches my hand hard.

"You don't have to say anymore, Bill. Somehow I knew."

I languish in the contact of his eyes. Finally. I bundle deeply in the presence of someone so near and dear to me.

In this instant there is heady mix of feelings. There is warm consolation and steamed resentment. I am angered at this grief. I want none of it. Not for my family. My aim is to get through this.

I hear my voice, measured and unnatural. "Bill, I have two questions to ask you. Are they going to take me back to the operating room soon to remove my uterus and, do I have less than three months to live?" His answer to each is, blessedly, no.

I have time! The thought seems to renew me. I have time to regroup and time to fight this monster inside of me. I will fight like hell. I like the sound of that. I like the strength I find it that. Norman Vincent Peale would be proud of me.

The aftermath of Bill's disclosure is relief. Mine, that it is done and Bill's, that the news does not destroy me. He calls the family into my room and they stand, side-by-side, like trees; strong, straight and lasting. I will need them. I will lean against them in the days and months to come. They are pained now and yet, reinforced by each other. Brothers and sisters. Such gifts to each other. "God, do not make me have to leave them."

"I will focus all in my power to overcome this disease," I say to them. "It is very important to me that you believe wholeheartedly that I will get better. I am determined to live every day of my life."

Each child hugs me, one by one. I watch the torment leave them. This is one more hurdle. There have been others and, God willing, there will be more.

The oldest son telephones late in the afternoon. He is away, out of state, and needs some positive assurance of my well being and my resolve. I wonder if they understood, all of them. I do intend to live, truly live, every day of my life.

In the beginning, when you are alone, fear has a chance to creep in on you.

Flakes of snow fall against the hospital window and I wonder. How many of my days ahead will be good ones? How many bad? What will the treatment be and how will it feel? You fear what you do not know.

The surgeon comes when my family is gone. He seems to clutch at the bottom of my bed like a warrior clutches at a shield. It is a barrier that he needs and I do not blame him for this form of self-protection. What strength would it take to close that barrier and how many times could he do it; day-in, day-out?

"I am sorry to tell you, you have cancer remaining in the pelvic area. We removed the mass and tumor, both cancerous, along with tissue invaded by cancer and some non-malignant tumor." He is matter-of-fact.

I learn that a band of scar tissue from previous surgery separates my stomach from the pelvic area and so my stomach was not biopsied. The results of biopsies performed were not good. Cancer was present throughout. An oncologist would visit me in a few days and a strategy will be mapped to fight the remaining cancer cells. Chemotherapy, radiation or both will be used. That decision remains with the oncologist.

My mind is strong. I know that now. I can cope with this. The unknown now is my body. How strong am I? How will I respond? Somehow I manage to ask this man, this surgeon, if there is even a chance that I can survive, or is this disease so far spread that I haven't even the slightest shot at recovery? I manage that and his response is measured, clinical.

"After all the biopsies are completed we will know what kind of cancer you have. Right now, we aren't sure what kind it is." I am confused now. I did know there were varieties of this disease. Later I learn that there are over 250 different kinds of cancer.

I tell him of my deep expectation; that I will beat this disease and recover. He smiles wanly and wishes me well. Not convinced, I think.

Radiation or chemotherapy. These new options to living sound unreal to me. Yet they are my options, for my life. Cancer is my reality and I am alone with these facts now, here in my hospital room.

Guilt comes. How could I have allowed this mutiny to happen to me? There must have been signs. How could I have ignored them? I know now that there were. Exhaustion late in the afternoon. My coping pattern of stretching across my bed for an hour or so each afternoon. My pelvis, always seemingly full but not distended. The luster of my eyes dimming. It seems peculiar now that I should remember thinking that my eyes were not the same. If I had taken these complaints to the doctor would he have recognized them? Questions.

Guilt erodes to a sinking resignation that maybe, for me, it is too late to battle this disease. I fight this fiercely and pray for the strength to maintain a positive lock on my attitude. I can feel how vitally important this is. Cancer is one more hurdle along my journey through this life. I know this intellectually and must work at knowing it viscerally.

Toward the end of that first day a candy striper pops in with a variety of floral arrangements. One of them is a dish garden of potted plants.

There is a small tag attached to the dish garden. "Guaranteed to last five years," it says. I laugh. Not bad odds; wish I had the same guarantee.

2.
Arming To Do Battle

a) A Spiritual Trio

b) Attitudinal Therapy

c) Meditation

d) Imagery

There are times in a man's life when,
Regardless of the Attitude of the body, the
Soul is on its Knees in prayer.

Victor Hugo

Another paradox about being seriously ill is how time treats you. While it seemingly takes itself from you it gives so much of itself for you to think. My initial hospital stay lasts nine days.

Survival too involves paradox. I must mesh iron will to out-of-hand acceptance. One extends from the other. I need to believe that indeed I will live. To do this I must accept whatever medical regimen is prescribed for me. I have to trust my doctors to do their part and trust myself to nurture my spirit. I am Catholic and I need all my resources now. Together we, the doctors, Padre Pio and me, can do this.

9

I believe in miracles and my soul is on its knees, now, in prayer.

I pray to Padre Pio to intercede on my behalf to the Sacred Heart of Jesus. This is merely my way. For others, people of other faiths, they will have their ways. This is mine.

I am a little girl on my father's knee. Whenever I pray for courage he is with me. He died twelve years ago. When I lay in the hospital bed he stays almost constantly on my mind. Daughters traditionally find strength in their fathers and I welcome him to my spiritual arsenal. My spiritual trio is formed: Padre Pio, the Sacred Heart and my Dad.

I look ahead. I plan. I plan for the future. For 'a' future. This is so vitally important. Planning is looking ahead to the future. Yes, I do expect to live.

Quality life? What is quality life...is every additional day of life, no matter how it is earned, not of some quality? The future will unfold and I will learn what it will be like in my struggle against cancer, and I must believe I shall be courageous in living, in meeting the challenges ahead.

Positive Attitude:

Norman Vincent Peale truly would be proud of me. I so believe that, for me, maintaining a positive vantage on my life is crucial. Make no mistake, I do not minimize. I have a disease that threatens my life. I do not reject the seriousness of my situation, but rather use a positive slant to grapple with the rigors of fighting this disease.

My reading on this topic is deep and varied. Indeed, I have made a study of biofeedback, biogenics. A whole library of layman's psychology has been scanned by me as I sunned on the beach or spent a sleepless night. It has been an avocation of sorts and I profit from it now.

My parents taught positive attitude to me. As an adult I take it on as a choice.

Early in my marriage I discovered a power. I can set the tone of my entire family. Indeed, in some strange way, I am the tone of my family. My mood becomes the prevailing wind and the course of our collective sailing is thus set. Surely each member of our crew had his or her time for thunder or squall and I was not exempt. But, my conscious determination was well worth the sacrifice. Keeping a bright eye on life sustained us through at least our share of pain throughout these years. It works.

I'll be strong now. You must remain in control of all the areas of your life for which you alone are responsible. You attitude is clearly within your control. I'll wax scholar here: Victor Frankl, in *Man's Search For Meaning,* told us that our last freedom is our freedom to choose the attitude with which we perceive our reality. Own this! The medical profession will use surgery, radiation and chemotherapy to save your life. You must be prepared to pick up the pieces medicine cannot handle.

Give yourself only a very little time to ask, WHY ME? if you must ask at all. And do not dwell on the suffering, on the assault against your body and your life. Negative thinking must not take command.

Meditation:

Prayer is talking to God. Meditation is listening. I learned this when my niece sent me a book on meditation based on the Edgar Cayce readings. It was all so new. I had to work extremely hard to familiarize myself with this discipline. There was nothing in my lifestyle to prepare me for meditation. I read and re-read the Cayce book, determined to absorb as much as possible. I can sense the worth in this. You learn the process of meditation at various levels of consciousness, the subconscious and the superconscious. Yes, this is all new but it need not be intimidating. Meditation is a valuable resource to me now.

Solitude, time, persistence and strong desire for serenity, inner peace and deeper relationship with God were what I needed to succeed at meditation. We've already discussed time. Cancer patients have lots of it. My family helped here. They allowed me to make myself my own top priority for the duration of this illness. Therefore I am able to master relaxation technique and retreat each day to collect my inner resources.

I possess strong faith and I make no claim here other than a simple statement of fact. My method of being and my method of meditation reflect my religious inclinations. I state this only to tell the reader that cancer is a human malady and knows no discrimination on any terms of division. This means that each must allow themselves their own reflection in meditation, imagery and so forth. My reflection took religious forms in the Sacred Heart, saying the Lord's Prayer and so forth. Please know that these are my reflections and I do not presume to prescribe them to anyone else.

Having attained the mental and physical point of preparation to enter into meditation, one is relaxed, free of outside influence and capable of spiritual indwelling. It is at this point that the readings of Cayce suggest that breathing exercises along with head and neck exercises should be performed. After the completion of this preparedness stage, I recited The Lord's Prayer, silently while concentrating on what are called the spiritual centers of the body, located in the endocrine system.

The initial part of the prayer is said concentrating on the pituitary, pineal and thyroid glands. The remaining part of the prayer is aimed at attunement with the gonads, adrenals, lynden and thymus. In stimulating these glands, a flow of energy is released to help achieve an affirmation. An affirmation is a tool for the mind used to build into our consciousness that which we seek to become. My affirmation is simple: "Let go and let God." This simple statement reflects my firm belief that God does want me to eventually be free of cancer.

Meditation cannot be forced. The goal is a state of spiritual, mental and physical harmony. Peace. I find that a great deal of patience is needed in meditation. A point of harmony is not always attained but, for me, meditation always brings relief from the nag of worry and a satisfying degree of relaxation. I am at peace. I have developed a new resource and a great source of spiritual communication.

Imagery:

Cancer is a revolt inside the body. Imagery creates a battlefield to help you fight back. I have read to imagine the good cells as soldiers inside the body, riding horseback and carrying spears. We send these soldiers racing through the body attacking the cancer cells. I do not find this image comfortable for me.

Instead, during meditation I imagine fluorescent light extending the width of my body. For me this light has a religious genesis. For me it is the healing light of Christ. The light starts at the top of my head and rolls slowly over my face: mouth, nose and chin. The slow rolling motion continues until it reaches the area of metastasis, my pelvis. Here I roll it back and forth, up and down, repeatedly. In my image it destroys the cancer cells as it rotates. I even feel a warmth; my light doing its life-saving work.

The illumination continues over the groin, thighs, legs, ankles, feet and extends through the toes, here departing the body. Imagery is part of my self-healing arsenal.

I want to do everything possible to help in the recreation of my body. My rebirth! My remission! My cure!

My desire to be cured. My trust in medicine and my belief that I am an active part of the healing process: these are the components that make my citadel. They all work in concert. (I write this twenty months after my initial diagnosis.) I know now that a diseased body does not obliterate peace of mind.

I was discharged from the hospital in March 1980. March is the promise of springtime. Perhaps March raindrops I see falling are tears of hope and tears of joy.

Only a precious few flowers survive to come home with me. The garden with the five year warranty thrives and sprouts. We go at it neck and neck.

3.
The Flower Show

I accept life unconditionally. Life holds so much—
so much to be so happy about always.
Most people ask for happiness on condition.
Happiness can be felt only if you don't set
conditions.

Arthur Rubinstein

The Philadelphia Flower Show. It truly heralds springtime in Philadelphia, my hometown. The Show is held in the famous rotund Philadelphia Civic Center and is an annual event for our family. My battle with the "Big C" would not do us out of this. I was determined.

This time I'd see the show on wheels! Bill called the Center and asked if we could get a wheelchair. We could. Bill and I, three daughters and a granddaughter went.

Touring the Show on wheels gave me a different perspective. It was curious to observe the public's response to a disabled person. At each display the crowd kindly gave way and I was wheeled to the front. My daughter threatened to leave me in a corner if I did not stop having such an unabashedly good time. She thought I should behave more invalid-like and less like someone enjoying the vantage of being in front of the crowd. We laughed. We had fun. We lived. We, quite literally lost control.

15

We were leaving and Bill pushed the wheelchair out onto the designated exit ramp. I looked down and suddenly felt an unmistakable acceleration. I glanced around to see Bill standing awestruck at the top of the ramp with two empty handle grippers in his now white knuckled hands. "Oh God no," he hollered, "Someone stop that wheelchair!" I picked up speed.

Options flashed upon me. Bail out and get run over by the damn thing or jerk the brake for all I was worth and go airborne. Decisions!

I heard sprinting sounds gaining fast. Suddenly two lithe bodies crashed into my lap. The extra weight of two of my daughters halted the wheelchair. We literally had to peel ourselves out of the chair we were laughing so hard.

I have cancer and yet I am having fun. I am alive.

Springtime of the year always makes me glad and grateful. Somehow I know that God will never call me home in the spring or the summer. Both these seasons are heavenly.

4.
Chemotherapy and Its Side Effects

Courage
Courage is the first of human qualities
because it is the quality which
guarantees all the others.

Winston Churchill

Even the word 'oncology' bodes stark and perhaps even evil. The word looks goat-legged. I fired the first one I met. I cannot tell you if this was a case of killing the messenger with bad news. At any rate, the man's manner brought with it no warmth nor even a stingy measure of assurance and I needed those feelings. I made my feelings known to my surgeon. A new referral was made and I was happier. Maybe I just needed the control, but if I were to make a partner of this person, this oncologist, I needed a more positive person and I am glad I was forthright and assertive. I was somehow convinced my actions were correct.

I shall tell you now of feeling fear, real fear; my first visit to the oncologist's office. This new oncologist had offered hope. I had ovarian cancer. That's what the biopsy told us. "Ovarian cancer sometimes responds favorably to chemotherapy drugs," he said. "In some instances

17

results are favorable." His words shimmered. Hope! White light! Possibilities! I stood now in this man's waiting room.

My stomach churns. No one should have to come this far and have no information, no counseling about what lies ahead. That unknown is precisely the core of my fear. It need not be. There should be someone assigned to do this. It is simply humane.

It is curious how fear distorts time and puts strange focus onto the simplest things we do. The signing of a form. The giving of a name. So pregnant with ambiguous meaning. I'll share the experience with you.

You sign a 'sign-in' sheet. The names of all patients who have been seen that day are on the sheet, in numbered sequence. It is important to remember what number you are in this sequence. I am number 21 this day.

The trick is to find this sheet. It has no designated place. It floats about the various rooms and must be found.

"You should go into the adjoining room and write your name on the yellow legal pad." I am an obvious neophyte and so another CA patient calls this information out to me as Bill and I enter the waiting area.

After we wait a seemingly endless time, a demanding voice calls out: "All numbers between 17 and 22 please come back." Back where? The voice had come from a young woman attendant who disappeared from the doorway where she made this announcement. I followed the others 'back there'.

Let me digress back to the patients in the waiting area. I was surprised. They were not particularly sad in appearance. Some were quite robust, others looked frail. A few men were partially bald and some of the women wore wigs. Two patients in particular stood out from the others; they were both terribly pale and quietly chatting about something called platinum. This substance would have lasting impression upon me later.

Once, 'back there' the following regimen takes place:

1. A sample of blood is drawn from a finger. The technician drawing it deposits it into three separate small vials. Later this will be studied under a microscope to determine a) white blood count, b) platelet cell count, c) hemoglobin, or red blood cell count. You get to pick which finger will be stuck.

2. You receive a physical directly from the oncologist. This is the only opportunity you will have to speak with him. You should have all your questions ready and be fully prepared to ask them. (Learn to talk fast if you want answers to all your questions.)

3. The chemotherapy drugs are injected intravenously, intramuscularly or both. Dosage is determined by the results of the blood sample. The circle is complete.

I am numbered therefore I am. I always abhorred the idea of being a statistic. I never dreamed it would happen so fast and take my identity with it.

I am benched and waiting my turn. 17, 18, 19 20...

I peer through the door at 20 getting her blood sample taken. "Twenty-one" is called. It is now MY TURN!

I have never been accused of acquiescence. The technician takes my blood and squirts it into three separate vials. Three vials times twenty-one patients is sixty-three vials of blood. I need no error made now. I approach the precipice. Dare I leap? From someplace deep within I hear my voice ask: "How will you keep an accurate identification of each patient's three vials of blood?" I pose the question in my best schoolgirl voice. Inquisitive, with deference. "Your number is on three of the vials," she says. I press. "I don't see number 21." She turns each vial to show clearly that, indeed, "#21" is neatly inscribed on each. I am relieved. Though I do not feel particularly popular.

The technician calls number twenty two. "You can leave," she says. Leave for where? I ask this of Twenty Two as we pass in the doorway. "You go back to the waiting room," he says. "And then they will call you in for a physical examination by the oncologist."

I am comforted talking with Twenty Two. He's been there, a vet. Naturally, instinctively I like Twenty Two. He lets me in on the KNOW.

I sit with Bill in the waiting area once more. Eventually a young woman calls my name, such a nice touch. I follow her into the examining room.

I am seated and alone. I am frightened again. God, I hope he will not give me more bad news.

If the world is turning at 33 1/3 rpms, I turn at 16 now. The oncologist is a 78. The door literally bursts open and this physician appears, talking quickly, moving fast. Not a second is wasted. No hesitation nor break in stride. "How do you feel Mrs. Quain"? He probes my abdomen. "Do you have any complaints?" I grade him in my mind. (Complaints, hell yes! First, I have cancer. Second, the coldness, disorganization and dehumanized toss and turn of this day and your office!)

"I'm anxious to know how long it will be before I am cured," I asked. He dances, he whirls. The oncologist deals with my directness with fleet-footed finesse. He reminds of the seriousness of having cancer. The seriousness that dictates my keeping up with this weekly regimen of chemotherapy for two years. (Which actually was a three year regimen.) He leaves.

While I put my clothes back on I understand.

Chemotherapy is a part of my life, for two years, each week. Alternative? Death. That is reality now and, today, I am number 21.

I return to the waiting room. Soon my number is called again. I return to the office area where bottles of drugs sit on a desk. I take two injections: one intramuscular, the other into my vein at the crux of my elbow. Gauze is placed over the injection sites. I am to sit in the office until the bleeding stops.

I would not want to work in this office. Surely they die a little each day. Surely, and yet, perhaps not. I play this out. I am assuming that they relate to us, we cancer victims, as people. Perhaps this cannot be so. I must then lose my identity here; at least for them. Each week I will return as some number between one and thirty. A statistic. Three vials of blood and two injection sites. A quick explanation of procedure, perhaps some consoling words from another cancer patient. I stopped! There is danger here. It's a deep, dark hole and not a grave, worse: self pity.

It really isn't up to this man, this oncologist if I am to be cured is it? It's a question of what God wants. He's in control now. He does his part. I do mine. The doctor does his. I am not alone here. I have my Spiritual Trio and I need them now.

Never say never. As I left the office I remembered a conversation I had with my sister three weeks prior to becoming ill. Never, we said, would we allow extreme measures to be taken to prolong our lives. Extreme has become such a relative term. Dylan Thomas shouts to me: "Do not go gentle into that good night. Rage, rage against the dying of the light."

Bill took me home. I will tell you now what chemo feels like. Bear in mind, it aims at a good; killing cancer cells. This fact must be born in mind.

An hour or so after injection exhaustion sprawls itself all over you. It drapes on you and weighs you down. It is relentless and conquering. It is not a myth. Chemotherapy takes a lot from you. Energy and appetite and even the will to conceal how you feel are gone. My stomach is a 'no man's land' and antacids replace food. An offensive taste takes over your mouth and sips of ice water slake your thirst and dilute this taste somewhat. The effects of these drugs leave no doubt about the vulnerability of the human frame against such a chemical onslaught. I am impressed.

By nightfall of the second day I can eat small portions of bland food. Pudding, bullion, jello. As days pass digestion improves allowing larger portions of these bland goodies.

I am too dependent on my family for my own tolerance. God bless them. They are here and willing to go in every and any direction.

5.
Solutions to Problems: Side Effects of Chemotherapy

"Your eyebrows are one shade darker than the hair on your head."

Anonymous

When I am feeling fitter it is time again for the next trip to the waiting room, to the numbered sequence, the physical and the injection of more drugs. I am on a treadmill now and the light, far off in the distance must be kept within my spiritual sight.

I am a veteran now. I know the ropes. I am familiar with the routine and that, at least, is good. You feel less disarmed. There is more control in knowing where the yellow legal pad might be. Confidence in the integrity of the three vials. Someone drives me to and from this place. We visit and I am without pretense, humbly human.

Weeks progress into months. I am wearied by this routine that weakens me as it seeks to save me. Days, each week are lost. I am abandoned to blinding exhaustion and a sickness of being that takes merely time to slowly remedy.

What am I being given? I need to know. That is my part in this and I will not allow it to be passive. My oncologist will not write the names of these chemicals for me. His penmanship is too far gone. "Tell me." He spells them out and I dutifully write them into my own note-pad.

Methrotrexate, adriomycin and fluoricil. These are/were the drugs. The year is 1980. Perhaps as the reader reads it is another time and there will be other chemical agents developed in this arsenal. But, at any rate, these are the drugs for me now. Later they will take stronger measures. We shall discuss that you and I.

Chemotherapy is a custom fitted regimen. Each type of cancer responds to different kinds of drugs. There are days when I receive no injection because my blood count is too low. A low blood count endangers one to infection. As my blood count drops I must take precautions against infections and other illnesses. Family and friends with colds elect not to visit so I won't catch their germs. I avoid large groups of people in closed rooms. I am determined to maintain acceptable health to continue chemotherapy. That too is part of my job.

On the pages following are suggestions that got me through the rigors of chemotherapy. No need to reinvent the wheel.

My aim here is to help people. I found these solutions to very nagging pragmatic difficulty after much frustration and a good deal of anxiety. Although I know that not everyone will experience the same side effects that I did I offer them here on the chance that someone else can benefit. I often thought that someone, in the hospital or the doctor's office could or should have told me what to expect and how to alleviate some of the misery. Perhaps no one had taken the time to compile a resource. Well, now we have a beginning. Perhaps I can make a contribution in this way.

(As I write this I am six months into my own bout with cancer.) I believe I am winning. It is taking its toll on everyone in my home. There is one exception though: the potted plant I took home from the hospital with me. It's doing great! A little greener, a little taller. New leaves sprout up. The florist guarantee card is on full display in the soil base.

I enjoyed the atmosphere of the working world, in addition to the responsibilities of homemaker and motherhood. However, the misdirected energy used in feeling sorry for myself that I no longer pursue previous activities drains me. It is obvious I will have to redirect my thinking and learn to accept the decreased energy level imposed upon me as a result of a stringent chemotherapy regime, and in particular learning to cope with the side-effects resulting from such powerful drugs.

"Cancer drugs cause two kinds of damage.* The drugs can make people feel very uncomfortable, with nausea, vomiting and diarrhea. Although patients really feel ill, we must remember that this discomfort is not a life-threatening condition. If the therapy will cure the cancer, then discomfort ought not to stand in the way of treatment, especially if the treatment will be given for a limited period.

The most dangerous side effects relate to renewing cell populations, especially in the bone marrow. There are different cells in your blood stream: white blood cells that fight infection, platelet cells that prevent you from bleeding, and red cells that transport oxygen. All these cells are produced in the bone marrow. Cancer drugs tend to prevent this production and result in a decrease in blood counts. Then there is a risk of serious problems; bleeding, uncontrolled infections and anemia. Experienced oncologists usually can avoid these problems by adjusting drug doses according to the blood counts. Dose modifications can prevent blood cells from decreasing to dangerous levels. Although oncologists can give these compounds with little risks of lethal complications, there are potential toxicities and patients need to understand them."

*"Medicine for the Layman," U.S. Dept. of Health and Human Services National Cancer Institute, NIH Publication No. 81-1807. Reprinted September, 1981.

There enters a new fight; the side effects of the drugs. Painful, annoying and frightening things start to happen to my body, countless and endless discomforts for which there must be some solutions. It seems obvious few solutions are available for the new problems, and generally this patient had to find solutions of her own. I will list here 'in a nutshell' some problems and solutions.

Problem #1: Nausea while going to and from the oncologist office.

Solution: Carry two small PLASTIC bags, one in your pocket or purse, the other under the seat of the car in which you are riding. Apprehension on the ride to the office and stomach distress following the chemotherapy injection leave me with uncertainty about how long I can control the nausea. It therefore seems logical to have the two plastic bags within easy reach.

Problem #2: Finding a driver to take you to the oncologist office for chemotherapy.

Solution: The oncologist attending me has offices at various locations, and on specific days of the week at each office. I chose Wednesday as my "chemo" day and selected the office closest to my home (approximately 20 miles distance). Therefore, family and friends are aware that Wednesday is a constant, and began to offer their services for a specific Wednesday of the month, taking turns with one another to do the driving. If you are not in this type of situation, there are drivers available through the American Cancer Society, driving patients to and from the oncologist's office, and in addition some community service organizations offer such services for a cancer patient. Do not overlook your church for volunteer drivers; it is important you contact someone associated with the church explaining your needs, because the church community may not be aware of this need for a driver unless you request it.

It took me approximately seven months before I felt secure enough to drive to and from chemotherapy. By the end of seven months a pattern begins; I do not become sick from the injection for a interval of one hour, and the exhaustion now sets in approximately two hours after taking the chemotherapy.

Problem #3: Can the nausea be prevented?

Solution: Ask the oncologist for medication which can be taken one hour prior to the injection. This can be an invaluable aid to lessen the spasmodic attack following chemotherapy injections. I learned this solution from another patient in the doctor's office. This person suggested I ask the doctor for some medication to be taken before the injection, and I did just that. He willingly wrote a prescription for a certain medication. This first medication was not effective and I asked for something else. He then ordered a drug named Vistaril, and this helped. I took this medication just before leaving my house, and it helped control severe nausea on most occasions. A point I want to bring out here is this: if I had not asked for some form of medication, it seems none would have been offered. Now I am convinced it is important I communicate all my needs to the doctor. I prefer asking for a prescription from the oncologist so that he will have a clear picture of what other drugs beside chemo I am taking.

Problem #4: Who can help you in finding solutions for your specific problem?

Solution: Sometimes the best self-help suggestions come from other cancer patients who have gone through the same concern you have. Or they will know of still another patient who had a similar problem to yours. And in this situation your family doctor is the best person to consult: he generally is aware of the side effects you may be experiencing and will offer advice. He too is more available than the oncologist. Yet I feel it is the patient's responsibility to keep each doctor informed of what drugs he takes so that there can't possibly be a counter-reaction of drugs in the system. If I am asked "is there anything that can be taken to help control nausea from chemotherapy?," I reply: "Ask the doctor for Vistaril." It is a wee bit of knowledge learned as a result of trial and error, and I happily share this information ONLY if asked.

Problem #5: Is the side effect experienced normal or expected?

Solution: Of course, ask the doctor first; but it appears oncologists have a great concern about cancer (understandable) and sometimes have little concern about common side effects. If the side effect is of genuine concern to the doctor, he will order specific tests to be done, or will ask the opinion of a specialist. The side effect you are experiencing may not be life-threatening in the overall picture, but it certainly can become almost intolerable to a patient. Again another cancer patient may have found a solution and relieve your concern that you are not the FIRST one to have such a reaction. Among cancer patients compassion exudes, and a tremendous willingness to help relieve worries of another, and in particular a novice patient, is never an imposition. Remember when you were in first grade and the eighth graders seemed so knowledgeable? So it is in this situation. One is a beginner and the other has weathered through many similar problems. Mostly you are in need of reassurance, and most side effects are temporary.

Problem #6: Will you lose your hair?

Solution: Again ask the doctor if the drugs you are taking will cause you to lose your hair. (Some drugs do not have this side effect and others do!) If his answer is yes, it does in some patients...be prepared! Once you experience the hair thinning (easily detected by examining the comb or brush you use and seeing lots of hair pulled away from the scalp) it is THEN you should find the location of a store specializing in wigs. Not necessarily even to go to the store but more importantly locating a place where a wig can be purchased when the need arises. If you wait until it is too late, all the hair may disappear and it will only add to your frustration if you don't know where you can purchase a wig. They ARE NOT sold in department stores in our area, where formerly they had been and where I believed they still were!

The hair of my head completely, completely disappeared in one week's time. Although it began to thin out a week prior, I believed there would be ample time to locate a wig before going bald. NOT SO!!! The baldness happened two months after I began taking chemotherapy.

After a few days' search, a wig store is found and here I learn that wigs can be matched in color to the eyebrows (if the head is bald, as in this case). The eyebrows are one *shade darker than* the hair of the head, I am informed. It is good I found a solution for my bald head when I did, because in a period of two weeks more I lost all the eyelashes and eyebrows.

The newly exposed scalp is not of the same texture as other areas of skin. It feels very much like a chamois, and of course is very white. The purity of the scalp and the loss of eyebrows and eyelashes makes me appear pale and sickly. I believe this is harder emotionally for my family to accept than it is for me. For them, I believe, it seems cruel that I am stripped naked of my former appearance, and they appear hurt that I am deprived of a natural complement—hair!!

I did not suffer psychologically with the loss of hair, as I had rather expected I would; but once I lost the facial hair, I began to dislike my looks. I do not feel I am slipping physically yet my appearance makes me appear fragile, and I hope the outward fragility does not attest to inward fragility.

Feel comfortable in asking another patient if he/she knows where a wig can be purchased. If the patient you ask is not wearing a wig, he will know someone in the office who is wearing one and get the answer you need from him. Once I purchased my wig I passed on the store's location and name to the oncologist's staff...it seems to me this information should be available through that office. The staff in turn referred other patients to me for this information. The American Cancer Society does not have this information available to patients and yet it seems it would. Another solution you must find on your own!

Problem #7: Some men are comfortable enough with the temporary baldness; however, if not:

Solution: Men's hairpieces can be purchased at a wig store which carries most styles in stock.

Problem #8: Is there an alternative for wearing a wig?

Solution: Purchase two or three cotton bandanas. Wigs sometimes become uncomfortable when worn for a few hours. In particular the pressure points securing the wig to a bald head become sensitive. Also wigs trap heat and the head becomes overly warm. The cotton scarf, tied gypsy style with the knot or bow at the nape of the neck, is quite acceptable and allows air to circulate through the cloth. I always wear the cotton scarf when in bed, since the wig is easily moved about when the head is on a pillow and again, the scarf is both more comfortable and cooler. Perhaps you might even be comfortable with a bald head while in the privacy of your home. If no one is at home, and I am not expecting anyone, I slip either the wig or bandana (whichever I am wearing) from the head and enjoy the freedom without something binding my head, but I always have either the bandana or wig in the same room with me, and in the event that someone comes I can easily cover the head.

I mention a cotton scarf, because all other materials tend to slip, are abrasive against the scalp, or trap heat. The good news is this: some patients experience thinning of the hair only, and others are bald for a short period before the hair starts to grow in again. I was bald for two years. It differs with each patient.

Problem #9: Can you adjust to the dependence on others as stamina decreases?

Solution: In the beginning of my illness I much resented my dependence on other people. Role reversal of mother and child annoyed and frustrated me, and yet the children are willing and supportive in every manner. Once it became apparent that my stamina and resistance went the way of chemotherapy devastation, another adjustment had to be made. I am no longer on the doing end in our home, but 95% on the receiving end. Therefore I MUST adjust to the weakened condition and reason that it is important for all of us that I not weaken myself further by overdoing in areas others can handle. Chemotherapy is making me better, I feel certain, and yet it also is weakening areas of my body. My legs in particular are greatly weakened and my arms seem to be losing strength. If I overexert myself I am aware of a shortness of breath. Physically I take care of myself, emotionally I feel the family and I offer each other strength and in most other areas the family does what needs to be done.

I adjust to being dependent on Bill and the children, along with help from my sisters and friends. I HAD to, and I DID!

Problem #10: The extreme of dependence?

Solution: When I felt well enough to go shopping, but too weak to walk any distance, a family member rented a wheelchair at the mall and willingly pushed me along past the stores where a purchase was to be made, and I waited in the chair while they did the shopping for me. Often I was buried by packages while seated in the wheelchair as we tried to accomplish as much shopping as we could, because the effort tired me and it was necessary to delay shopping for any length of time or in the near future. However the outing is refreshing always!

Problem #11: Mouth ulceration. There sores are difficult to endure, and so bothersome at times that it is difficult to eat or drink. Although I suffered this side effect, many other "C" patients do not experience the same reaction.

Solution: When the ulceration is severe enough the oncologist stops treatment for awhile to allow the tissue to heal enough to allow food and drink intake. When the ulceration is more than moderate and almost more than tolerable, a prescription called Xyocaine Viscous Solution can be ordered which when applied temporarily numbs the mouth allowing the patient to eat and drink.

On one occasion the oncologist responded to ulceration in my mouth with this statement: "It's a good sign really, while chemotherapy is producing sores in the mouth it also is attacking the live cancer cells in your body in the same manner." His statement certainly didn't help much. Although I understood his philosophy, I adhered to my psychology. It was figuratively and literally hard to swallow! *Added solution:* TRY NOT TO HIT THE DOCTOR!

Problem #12: Tissue sensitivity of the mouth. The tissues of my mouth are always sensitive now, even after the ulcers disappeared. Therefore many alternatives must be developed to help me eat and drink enough substance to prevent a great weight loss.

Solution: A straw! Straws are placed within easy reach at my bedside and in the kitchen and bathroom. When drinking through a straw, I can position it far back in the mouth letting the liquid bypass the lips and damaged tissues of the mouth passing directly to the throat.

THESE ARE UPSETTING TIMES FOR MYSELF AND FAMILY DUE TO THE LOSS OF WEIGHT THAT NATURALLY ACCOMPANIES LIMITED EATING.

Problem #13: What replaces toothpaste once the mouth tissues become sensitive?

Solution: Once the tissues inside the mouth became sensitive, brushing with toothpaste causes a burning sensation. Warm water and salt are used instead of toothpaste both for brushing the teeth and as a mouthwash to help ease soreness. When there is an offensive taste in the mouth (side effect of some chemotherapy drugs) this solution is equally helpful. An alternative method is to brush or rinse the mouth with baking soda and warm water. The salt and warm water have a healing effect. The oncologist on one occasion prescribed a mouthwash, but it was not as soothing as the above mentioned, so I stayed with the more effective solution.

Problem #14: Weight loss.

Solution: At one point it is obvious that the doctor believes I need to add a few pounds, and he suggests a hearty milkshake combination of: 1) milk, 2) one egg, 3) a healthy portion of ice cream, 4) a little whiskey (for calories). He advises three milkshakes a day as a substitute for meals I am missing due to pain (ulceration). Of course I will use the all important straw to drink with. One VERY FILLING MILKSHAKE was digested and I slept for a long, long nap; approximately four hours later my daughter awakened me to say I had slept the entire afternoon. Tenderly she suggested that perhaps I was a little heavy-handed with the whiskey portion of the milkshake!!! I continued with the three (3) milkshakes daily, omitting the whiskey portion, and did regain some of the lost weight.

Problem #15: Dryness of the mouth. Some chemotherapy drugs cause severe dryness of the mouth lining and tongue, which results in a frequent and insatiable thirst. This isn't a particular problem when at home because ice and water are readily available, but if there is going to be a significant time lapse before a liquid can be had, then a solution has to be found.

Solution: Traveling away from home I carry a thermos of ice water in the car along with a straw. Hence the thermos becomes a constant companion and generally is drained of its contents when I reach my destination. At this point in my illness icewater is a favorite traveling drink, for more than one obvious reason; aside from being refreshing there is no worry about spoilage. In other areas away from home water fountains are available and I choose water and ice as a drink when visiting, as I am now certain it will not cause an upset stomach.

Problem #16: Other digestible liquids?

Solution: Other suitable liquids for a sensitive mouth and/or the "great thirst," are: milk and iced tea, which (for me) replace all sodas and hot drinks because heat or carbonated beverages cannot be tolerated. Milk and iced tea are soothing and replenish lost fluids in the body. Gatorade (the athletes' drink) is a healthy and palatable drink. As a matter of fact both the oncologist and physicians suggest I drink Gatorade while I am in the hospital, and when my strength is weakened on other occasions. It not only relieves thirst but replaces electrolites in the system. Only the orange flavor Gatorade is well tolerated (by me) and other flavors are not purchased because they failed the taste test. I drink at least three glasses of Gatorade daily and always place a glass of Gatorade or ice water at bedside taking sips upon awakening from thirst.

Problem #17: Is there a substitute for water when one is neither in a car (with thermos) or near a fountain or at home?

Solution: A Fannie May orange lollipop. The lollipop will activate the saliva glands bringing moisture in the mouth. I can often be seen with a taffy stick protruding from my lips, and am no longer embarrassed about what people will think seeing a grown woman with a lollipop in her mouth. I mention the brand Fannie May because most other brands are too tart (although if the mouth is in a normal condition you are not aware of this). I also mention the orange flavor lollipop is far superior to hard candies, because it can be removed readily from the mouth by the stick, whereas hard candy is sticky when removed by the fingers, and at frequent intervals. In addition while in the mouth, the hard candies can bump against ulcerated tissue (if present). A committee of one, me, recommends a lollipop be carried in pocket or purse for a quick and pleasant temporary relief of thirst, or offensive taste of the mouth.

People's reactions seeing me with a lollipop stick protruding from the mouth are often amused. I was shopping with my husband and a passerby grinningly remarked "You're only a kid at heart, aren't you." We laughed. He never knew what a therapeutic effect a lollipop can be to a chemo patient.

Problem #18: What other foods are palatable when the appetite is poor, or the mouth sensitive?

Solution: My diet always consisted of bland foods of soft consistency. (I would have killed for a piece of toast at breakfast, but it has sharp edges, did you know? If your mouth is sensitive you know!)

Hotcakes helped satisfy my hunger at many a meal, and for any meal. Eating less food at more frequent intervals seems to help keep me from losing too much weight. (During my illness I lost 20 lbs., going from 119 to 99 lbs.) When I discovered hotcakes were digestible I also found the convenience of frozen batter to be a perfect solution in preparing hotcakes for one person. Simply defrost and pour out the desired amount of batter to be cooked. Tapioca and rice puddings satisfied my appetite, along with mashed potatoes and rice flavored by chicken bouillon gravy. Limitless portions of vanilla ice cream also appeased my hunger.

Beef and chicken bouillon cubes made into broth made an easy and nourishing meal (let the broth cool to room temperature before eating and don't forget the straw!). The bouillon also supplemented lack of sodium.

Problem #19: How to help ease the pain in the legs while confined to bed?

Solution: After a time on chemotherapy my legs were both painful and lacking strength, so I generally slept with a pillow underneath the back of the knees, easing discomfort. While sitting I generally propped the legs up on an ottoman which also eased strain.

6.
Stress and Natural Immunity Theory

Did I give myself cancer? Did I bring it on myself? Do I deserve it?

There is a medical theory stating that through embracing stress in our lives, we damage ourselves. As for me, and I believe, most people; I was just busy living. Stress was purely secondary.

Stress induced disease. I don't buy it. I don't need to add responsibility for my developing cancer to the already awesome task of fighting it.

I mention this because there is one responsibility we must embrace. Putting the stress we must deal with in perspective. We need to understand that the same positive imagination that develops the thought of internal warriors fighting cancer can also become destuctive. Deal with reality. Don't inflate possibilities beyond the situation in which you find yourself.

My message is this: minimize stress. If you have a pain, talk about it to your doctor. Having the diagnosis of cancer seems to make every anatomical twinge significant when it may not be. Do not allow yourself to fantasize. Tell the doctor and bring your concern to the light of day. It is what you do not know, but worry about that can harm you. I was diagnosed with rheumatoid arthritis just four months prior to the diagnosis of cancer. But now, when I experienced pain in my left leg I toyed with all the possibilities and the ramifications and this volley began to wear on me. I finally confessed to my doctor that I was afraid of mentioning the pain yet I knew that medical assurance was the only remedy for my trepidation. You don't have to go through that.

Again, I am most uncomfortable with the notion that I could have avoided having cancer. The only control is diagnosis early enough to do battle, and the physical strength to withstand required treatments.

Having a large family taught me that there is camaraderie and warmth that develops from need. Three of my children have severe vision limitations. They are, in fact, legally blind. Another child is a diabetic and has fought long and hard with this disease.

My point here is this: We rallied together yet each stood alone. Even with optimum support each person's anatomy reacts to some degree. There is no escaping this. All we do is minimize the effects and remember that even loving someone brings a certain degree of stress to our lives. Caring costs; it is part of being alive.

In analyzing current theories about stress induced cancer I can merely say that it seems incongruous that devastation should bring with it further devastation. I hope that authors on the topic will avoid pointed innuendo stating that cancer patients have somehow failed themselves and allowed stress to have its way with them, lessening their immunity to disease and have therefore played an active part in their own demise. One thing people fighting cancer do not need is guilt.

I conclude that we do well in preparing ourselves to deal with stress. Now that I have a very real physical disability I embrace my natural combatants: Faith, attitudinal therapy, imagery and meditation. In a stressful world, response, not exposure seems key.

7.
And The Bills Just Keep Coming...

.....and the bills keep coming! The pragmatics of any disease, let alone a lengthy illness, demand that someone must keep a record of expenses. It seems inappropriate to equate expense with illness, but they do go hand in hand, and the responsibility of keeping track of the expenses depends upon the patient or another family member. I elected me! Paradoxically, being severely ill made me an excellent bookkeeper as I developed an accurate and concise method of filing bills and keeping up-to-date records of what has been paid and what bills are still outstanding. I don't pretend even to hint this is always easy to do, nor would I trick you into believing I often felt up to such a task. The task though is simplified by using the methods described here:

1) Purchase a copybook.

2) Buy a small supply of 5 x 7 envelopes, along with a large rubber band.

3) On the first ruled page label your name e.g. Kay's illness.

4) On this page also list the name, address and telephone number of each doctor treating you for this illness.

39

5) Turn page and secure this page with the rubber band over and also over the front cover of the copybook.

6) As doctor and hospital bills arrive store these bills under the rubber band, which will be the page on the left side of the double page.

7) When you feel well enough to concentrate proceed by placing information from the bills in column form on the right hand page opposite the rubber band held page.

8) At the top of the page where you are listing the information contained on the bills label the top of the page—CLAIM #1.

The listing in these columns should coincide with the bills filed between this page and the preceding page (held by the rubber band). The heading CLAIM #1 is for your bookkeeping records only, and should not be submitted with your payment of bill. After all the bills recorded on this page have been paid, take same bills and place in 5 x 7 envelope (mark on envelope CLAIM #1), and file in a safe place in a easily reached area. I kept my copybook with due bills in a tote bag in the closet of my bedroom, both out of the way and easily accessible for me when I felt well enough to do the bookkeeping. In this way you have a record of all bills in two forms; one written in the copybook, the other the actual bill itself stored in the envelope.

Once you have completed paying the bill entered on CLAIM #1, turn to the next double page and move the rubber band forward to hold this new page over the preceding page. Mark the right hand page CLAIM #2, and keep records of all new current bills now stored behind the rubber band, entering new information exactly as registered on the page marked CLAIM #1.

INFORM A FAMILY MEMBER OF YOUR METHOD OF BOOK-KEEPING AND TELL HIM WHERE YOU ARE KEEPING THE COPYBOOK AND PAID BILLS. This way someone can continue to keep records for you should you become too ill to continue.

Should you have to submit bills to an insurance company, make a copy of the original bill and mail that to the insurance company, keeping either the original or copy for your records. NEVER MAIL ORIGINAL WITHOUT RETAINING A COPY.

If your bills are paid by the insurance company directly to the doctor or hospital, you will receive a notice from the company showing what amount was paid and to whom. Mark that payment in your book beside the recorded bill.

A procedure of some insurance companies is to send the money directly to you. The responsibility is then yours to pay outstanding bills, reimbursed by insurance company.

AFTER ALL BILLS REGISTERED ON PAGE MARKED CLAIM #2 have been paid, remove copies of bills and place in envelope (mark envelope CLAIM #2) and file away with previous claim in the same designated storage place. Now you have a genuine cross file of all bills paid. Continue in sequence for the remainder of illness.

Keep all drug bills for prescriptions. If they are reimbursed by an insurance company, make copies, send originals to the insurance company, and retain the copy for your records. DRUG BILLS ARE NOT COVERED BY BLUE CROSS OR MEDICARE. (1980)

All expenses paid by you and not reimbursed may be totalled on your income tax return as medical expenses for that year. Therefore record keeping is important!

If you are eligible for Medicare and the doctor's office does direct billing, Medicare may pay the doctor directly, sending a statement of the payment to you.

If the doctor's office DOES NOT do direct billing to Medicare, you are responsible for paying the doctor (or hospital) and you in turn submit the bill to Medicare (be sure to make a copy of the bill before sending it!!!).

Medicare will pay you directly and you are responsible for payment to the doctor (or hospital).

Should you have Medicare and Blue Cross 65 Special, bills should be sent to Medicare by either the doctor's office or by you (as described above). The balance not paid by Medicare should be automatically billed to Blue Cross 65 Special. Records of all bills paid by both Medicare and 65 Special will be mailed to you. KEEP THEM, FILE THEM.

IF YOU ARE NOT CLEAR ON ANY PROCEDURE CALL THE COMPANY WITH WHOM YOU HAVE INSURANCE, AND BE PERSISTENT IN ASKING QUESTIONS UNTIL YOU HAVE A SATISFACTORY EXPLANATION.

If you are too ill or it's too complicated, perhaps someone close to you—family, friends will help. There's no harm in asking.

I am a firm believer in medical insurance and know that a catastrophic illness such as cancer can destroy a family financially. Given the chance to advise others I would caution them carefully to review medical insurance options. Personally, I feel that National Health Insurance should be initiated to cover ALL catastrophic illnesses. I am fortunate that my longstanding belief in insurance sustained us financially. I do not feel I could have withstood the worry of depriving my family of their needs because of my immediate need. We would, of course, have had to meet that challenge, but I was spared that worrry, thus alleviating additional stress.

October 14, 1981...

...Nightime works a magic upon insomniacs...I am Henry Higgins crooning to Liza Doolittle; "My Fair Lady." She is transformed into a glass of water on my night table... "I've grown accustomed to the glass...(I take license)...it simply makes the thrist grow dim...I was serenely independent and content before we met" ....magic or madness. And I have grown accustomed to the "glass," placed each night, full of water and ice, by some family member. A duty of love, made a ritual for me and most appreciated.

I have to undergo more surgery and I haven't told anyone. I keep it to myself and I don't really know why just now. If I told them would I now be less restless? I reach out for the glass of ice water. It hits my mouth with welcomed force against the cracked dryness.

The concept of moistness takes me to the leaf drying on my chest of drawers. Drying in the night. I fight off the lyrics of yet another night-crazed tune and laugh at myself. It helps stave off the knife play of fear in my stomach. More surgery. More surgery and cis-platinum chemotherapy treatments. I am alone and I am afraid this night and I cling, with just a hint of desperation, to my Spiritual Trio.

8.

Cis-Platinum* Treatments

Resurgence
Out of the earth, the rose,
Out of the night, the dawn
Out of my heart, with all its woes
High courage to press on.

Laura Lee Randall

Prologue

Even writing this is hard for me. It, the writing, brings memories reeling back upon me. They are green-monstered child memories that wake one in the night, terrified and alone. I had six treatments, all given as an inpatient over a period of seven months. Remembering this time makes me nauseous, one of the side effects of cis-platinum.

*PDR: *Platinol, Cis-platin, Cis-diamminedichloroplatinum;* generally referred to as: cis-platinum treatments, and so used in this book.

45

And so writing, this writing, is therapeutic. I hope it will be cathartic and rid me of more delayed response.

Cis-platinum is needed to prolong my life. Tolerating repeated treatments is difficult because the first one hammers hard and unrelenting. Willingness to do it again is obliterated. And yet one must.

Two notions saw me through this time: Reactions to the drug are temporary and discomfort decreases; remission is the hoped for light at the end of the tunnel.

My telling the story now is not an attempt to discourage one who may be faced with this alternative. The fact that I am here to tell it is, perhaps, the most compelling testament for its taking.

The news that this chemotherapy would mean that I would be in the hospital again disheartened me. I had not counted on this. My oncologist was frank about the effects of cis-platinum. While I would not have had this any other way, his frankness challenged me, and weighed my spirits. "Are the treatments necessary?" I felt my shoulders droop. My spirit sagging.

"If you were my wife," he said, "I would certainly want you to go ahead with cis-platinum treatments."

My doctor explained that ovarian cancer is often responsive to this drug.

"You will be mad at me for a few days," he said. "Cis-platinum causes severe nausea lasting as long as twenty-four hours after injection."

My mind shot back to the oncologist's office waiting room, months ago. There were two people, frail, pale and with skin nearly transparent. In hushed tones they spoke of cis-platinum. I had singled them out because of their appearance. Their chalk skin made a mockery of my summer tan.

I made the decision to go with the treatment as added armor. The treatments started two weeks after my doctor's notification and this interval is marked by deep anxiety. I fight this.

I learn that the patient's tolerance for the treatment determines the length of the hospital stay. Mine lasts seven days.

Cis-platinum was discovered in 1960. It is administered according to body weight. Anywhere from 30 to 160 milligrams is given. The patient must be hydrated before and after administration.

The procedure begins with a creatinine test, determining kidney function. This clearance takes the first twenty-four hours of the hospital stay.

One of the most serious side effects of this treatment is kidney damage. Platin by-product is a metal that could damage the kidneys. With blood tests completed, a "go-ahead" is given.

Intravenous needles are inserted and the saline hydration begins. This continues for many hours.

A chemotherapeutic drug called Bleomycin is dripped for twenty-four hours and massive quantities of diuretics are given orally to the prepare the kidneys for the cis-platinum solution. This final step takes thirty minutes to one hour. With tubes and needles still in place the onslaught begins.

Allow me a humorous side note. Bill came to visit me early the afternoon of my first treatment. I had had Bleomycin and mistakenly supposed it to be cis-platinum. I explained that, much to my gleeful surprise, I had avoided the dreaded wretching. I was impressed with my resistance to the powerful drug.

Later in the day I was stunned when the cis-platinum hit my system. My resistance was shattered. The nausea persisted for a full five days.

It is not possible to describe the effect of this drug. You are thoroughly washed out. You lose control of your bladder because of the diuretics. The wretching continues beyond anything you might have imagined and it drains you. Your energy is gone and the hours, to go through this internal destruction, linger.

Kay Quain ceased to exist for a time under this assualt. I could utter no response and my blood pressure plummeted. I lose consciousness and go into shock. I am frightened. Through this my hearing comes and goes. I hear that my pressure is dropping. The voice saying this is on the edge of panic and now I am too. I cannot take myself up and over the edge of this chemical. I am in deep trouble and have no way of responding.

If you are a clinician reading this book please know that patients can hear you in the most seemingly dire of situations. Discussions about conditions should be held away from patients, or, at least, in hushed tones. To be without the wherewithall to respond and to be frightened is a special kind of hell.

Beyond this experience, I look upon the second cis-platinum treatment with untold trepidation. I am scheduled to re-enter the hospital in another four weeks for the second treatment.

Meditating is my solace now and yet it has never been so difficult for me. I use imagery. I place myself, sitting, by the side of the sea. I find peace here and this helps me soothe my body through my mind.

This trauma comes again in November. When I return from the November treatment a new malady comes upon me. The soft tissue on the inside of my mouth has literally peeled away. This is a side effect of Bleomycin. I attempt to disguise this but the discomfort wins. I am in agony. Eating and drinking were not possible. I say to Bill, "Do you know water has sharp edges?"

A druggist friend suggest that my doctor prescribe Xylocaine Viscous. It works! The effect is to numb the inside of my mouth. I am able to drink. Teaspoons of cool water are sheer pleasure.

I must tell patients that another responsibility they must develop is telling physicians the extent of pain they feel. Why did my druggist have to tell me about Xylocaine? I had told my doctor the pain I felt; had I not been convincing enough? Be firm in describing what you feel.

Following the November treatment I was sedated and confined to bed for another week after I left the hospital.

I know that I must fight this weariness. It seeks to beat me. I cannot be passive with my complaints. The thought that I will have to go through this again in 18 days appalls me. I face it. Psychologically I am now frightened!

With the third treatment in December I again lapse into unconsciousness. Tests discover that a sodium deficiency is the culprit. I increase sodium intake and the problem is corrected.

My doctor tells me to eat food higher in sodium content. He suggests potato chips and pretzels. I remember the nausea and the condition of my mouth. I just smile. Sometimes the loneliness comes at you in the strangest ways and is precipitated by the oddest of events. Not even my doctor really understands what chemotherapy does to someone. To me.

In December I leave the hospital after five days. My treatments are half over. The kids send a bouquet. "Hooray, Mother, you have reached the halfway mark!" I am able to embroider Christmas stockings in the hospital.

Simple things like reading and embroidery mean a lot. I take these signs that come with the December hospitalization to mean I am getting stronger.

The family is able to ignore my sallow complexion and the Holidays are a blessed reprieve from the battle that wants to consume everything within my life. The new stockings are distributed. Gifts are exchanged. Talk never touches my illness and I am grateful.

I find a new wrinkle on New Year's Eve. We had dinner at a friend's home and as usual we talked endlessly. When it came my turn I got three sentences out and was totally short of breath. I could not continue! The slack in the conversation was picked up effortlessly by a friend, but Bill and I opted to leave early.

My shortness of breathe was new and disturbing. I could not walk up steps without stopping. Telephone conversations were labored. My doctor orders a Gallion scan. This involves radioactive contact medium being injected into the circulatory system and followed through the lungs. It finds a lack of elasticity in my lungs, fibrosis. Bleomycin is deemed the culprit and discontinued.

Peripheral neuropathy has developed in my fingertips and both feet. This is caused by the chemotherapy. Doctors tell me it may be temporary. Again, no guarantees. When the chemo is finished we'll wait.

The third, fourth and fifth months of cis-platinum unfold with their terrible debilitation and parallel hope for salvation. I implore my family and friends not to visit me in the hospital. It distresses me to see their faces as they respond to my fight and helplessness. My family does not relent. They visit me every day.

I must tell you that it takes virtually every once of resolve to continue with the remaining treatments. They seem to take me close to death itself. My veins are in a state of collapse for the remaining treatment. The IV-team probes for a suitable site.

The spring of 1981 brings with it beauty and the last of the six cis-platinum treatments. I am weak beyond telling. During this time people have told me they would not have taken these treatments. I think perhaps they would behave differently if they truly had to face my options. There is the possibility of a remission. You must take it.

To those who face cancer I must relate the legion of emotions I deal with. These emotions come at you strong. They mix and flare and flicker. There is the steel-strong will to continue living. There is life, life with suffering and the conflicting push to have it continue. One must face oneself in the mirror and face what one sees. This is very hard sometimes. You watch your family watch you. You watch them wonder about your death and about your life and your will to live. You love them and yet, almost in paradox you wish desperately for privacy with yourself and your suffering and doubt and pain. Above all of this there is the will to hinge your mind onto some interest outside of this disease and this suffering. This is a discipline with which you have fleeting success.

These are the goblins that gather and go one year into this regimen called chemotherapy. Yet, there is a strength in this. I am a veteran; part of an elite. A pioneer. Yes, and stronger now. I am alive. I am surviving cancer.

9.
The Medical Profession

Forgive me if too close I lean
My human heart on thee.

John Greenleaf Whittier

He wears roller skates! I know he does. My oncologist seems to materialize and then disintegrate in and out of my hospital room. I move toward him and he is gone. I practically fall from my bed. I speak fast but he moves faster. I have unanswered questions and he has other patients to see.

If my oncologist got paid by the word he'd starve.

He is inside his exam room firing pleasant economical greetings as he moves. In a motion his hands probe the site of my surgery. He is pleased. He says "you're doing fine" as he pats my back and moves toward the door. Gone! At best I can catch him poised, hand on doorknob. His hand operates the mechanism as the question is answered. Gone! He is water through rock. Remarkable!

Seventeen patients are examined and treated in two and a half hours. Although my questions upset the movement of this clock, I persist: What

53

is the course of my treatment? What drug is being administered? What are the side effects? What do my symptoms mean?

I insisted on answers in layperson's terms when their jargon confused me. After months of this the oncologist got the message. This lady wants to know everything that is happening to her.

Trust is a bridge, and it must be built upon solid information. Trust is vital for the patient to give him or herself over to the oncologist. The stake is life. The holder of the information is the physician. The one in need of this information is the newly diagnosed cancer patient. The course of the transaction is clear.

I noticed yet another paradox. As my trust developed over the months of treatment, the terse nature of the oncologist softened. Perhaps I was projecting. Perhaps my own initial lack of trust translated into a misperception on my part. Perhaps the point is mute. Patients need information. They are apprehensive and information begins to alleviate this.

I wonder if oncologists and oncology nurses must consciously steel themselves against the agony of patients being battered by the side effects of chemotherapy. Perhaps this is the only way they can continue to do what they do. To partake of so much suffering might just be too much for anyone. I can understand that. I can say, though, that when I understood, when I received the information I sought, treatment became a little more bearable.

I mistrust ego. I trust my doctor because he never allowed ego concern to cloud his science. I felt this. Whenever a new development concerned him he referred to a specialist. He never pretended to have all the answers. I trusted that in him. He was a human being and sometimes "all too."

There were six of us sitting in the waiting room. The inner door burst open and my doctor's face was crimson. "You were told to enter the hospital yesterday. That could not have been made more clear to you." He unleashed these words on a patient sitting there.

His anger was crystal clear and the experience upset all of us. I believed it was unnecessary to subject everyone to this verbal outburst and told him so behind closed doors.

I need to explain what it means to be frail. You are brittle. You are truly buffeted by the wind. Sound assaults the mind. Cold takes you over. Anxiety clutches you with long-nailed, bony fingers as you sit waiting for the injection of a toxic chemical into your bloodstream. You do not need to witness the verbal execution of a compatriot. When it came my turn in the examination room I unloaded. I summed by saying if I were to be the recipient of a reprimand it would happen in private, between us, behind closed doors.

The doctor, I think, let his armor down for just a moment. I know I heard it hit the floor. His response was, again, all-too-human. "I simply could not believe anyone would want to jeopardize their life that way."

The patient's condition was near critical. The doctor was genuinely concerned.

The emotional interplay between patient and physician is an intricate lacework. Through it all there are times of great compassion felt through a maze of tubes, vomiting, gut wrenching, body twisting spasms. There are times when you need something human and, instead, you are made pain-fully aware of the physician's need to insulate him or herself from you and your legion of fellow sufferers. The effect is to isolate the patient, me, my fellows. I resent this but understand it. I'll go further: this isolation is not healing. It is the cold shoulder. A cowardice. Death. It does nothing positive but allow the physician, the nurse, whomever, the space to do all of this again tomorrow. Again, I understand it.

It was about 11:15 PM one night. I was awake in my hospital room watching local news and three young nurses tapped on the door and then peeked their heads in. Could they come in? "Of course," I said.

I was asked a question that told me many things. The question was: "how could a nurse better help a cancer patient?" The question had side-bars too: "what were my true feelings about the disease, the treatments, the side effects?"

What the question told me was that there was a gap in the education of these nurses. They were clinically competent. Yet their education stopped at compassion, or, more precisely, at empathy. However, it was their genuine reaching within themselves, and their courage to stretch who they were that brought them to my bedside that night. That is what really burned brightest for me.

I told them what I know and what I felt. I also felt a great deal of pride for them. I expressed by admiration to them for asking direct questions of a cis-platinum patient. I only hope that what I told them would reap benefits as they went forward in their profession. I was impressed by them that night and will never forget them.

I must make a point here. Chemotherapy involves needles. Lots of them! They pierce your arms and your hands, always in search of a vein: a port of entry. Your veins deteriorate and then it takes a pro to search your arms, to search hands, to find a vein. I cite this because, realizing that clinicians need to practice to get good, cancer patients are big league. No place for sandlotters. I would counsel anyone to make this point with their physician. It is an outrage to endure someone who does not know, or worse, does not care, jabbing an already insulted body.

I have an observation. Any person who I have regarded as great, usually had within him or her some strong strain of humility. This observation holds for doctors, too. They are not gods. The best ones know it. They are instruments through which His Will is accomplished. Again, the best ones know this.

Yet, I must get this venom out. Please get in line: doctors, residents, interns, nurses, technicians. You are blessedly few, but the insensitive ones deserve this. To borrow some of your phrases: 1) "This won't hurt." 2)

"You'll feel a little stick from the needle, that's all..." 3) "You may experience a slight burning from the dye,..." (I seared inwardly)... 4) "That is not a known side-effect..." 5) "I don't know why you feel this way..." 6) "We lost the sample you gave us, Kay. If you'll just give us another the results will only be a few days late..." 7) "If you have any complaints call me," (I can't reach him for four days)... 8) "Aspirin should help..." (I need morphine, not aspirin)... 9) "What you are experiencing will only last a week..." (I hope I last a week).

There is a message behind this litany. Each was actually part of my medical experience. Each was uttered in condescension and raised my hackles.

I must object, too, to the objectivity with which one is regarded by so many practitioners. Conversations are held right over you. You are not included. Identity wanes and waxes as the doctor strips you down to room number, weight, temperature and an assorted array of bodily functions. One is probed, hands and arms and legs are raised and lowered upon command.

Questions are shot at you. Hundreds! Yet not once was I asked if I was under any stress aside from my disease. Fifty years count for not one thing! I am a statistic! A disease entity! I have no mind anymore, at least not one that a physician will address.

A physician's time is limited. I know that. How about my time? My life might be ticking away here. Give me a few minutes for God's sake, if not for mine. I am a living human being. At least for now. You give me a total of six to eight unencumbered minutes. Minutes for which I pay dearly.

The doctor and the patient should be partners. In an imperfect world, one where people still got cancer, wouldn't this be the best possible relationship? I realize they must insulate themselves from all the pain if they are to keep on healing. I reject, however, the idea that the healer's insulation should isolate the patient. Having cancer is hard enough without that.

Listen to what it is like to have this disease. I will tell you. But, again, you could ask a human being to tell you what she feels. What her skin feels like when her veins are all collapsed. What her mouth feels like when the lining is gone and water feels like glass. What the shock is like when you put your hand to your head and there isn't any hair. What it feels like and what you fear when the woman you've befriended in the oncologist's waiting room is not there anymore.

All of these fears and twinges are the feelings wrought by cancer. Yes. But they are also wrought and processed by fifty years of living on this earth. Those years matter too. I am a human being!

Allow me these rejections: 1) I recoil and retreat from a rebellious professional. 2) I am strengthened by clear, concise communications with a physician. 3) I object to brittleness on the part of anyone associated with medicine. 4) I have no time for a health professional bringing the contagion of his bad humor with him or her to work.

Physician, heal thyself.

10.
Family Adjustment

There's a special king of closeness
That only families know,
That begins with childhood trust
and deepens as you grow.

There's a special kind of happiness
in sharing little things,
The laughter, smiles, and quiet talks
that daily living brings.

There's a special kind of comfort
in knowing your family's there,
To back you up, to cheer you up,
to understand and care—

Of all the treasures life may bring,
your family means the most,
And whether near or far apart
that love will hold you close.

—Author Unknown

Aside from the assault on your body by cancer, there is something else. This new hurt to contend with is created by the fact your newly disabled condition is not your pain alone, but is shared by family and friends. I realize only too well their doubts, and they, in their love of me, were being caused a great deal of suffering.

I can't go this route alone, I know, and yet how can I share my anxiety and pain? How much shall I share my thoughts and fears? These are questions for which there are no established answers.

A schedule is developed around my times of exhaustion—ah! so willingly—and flexibility permeates the air; routines are ignored; rigid schedules are set aside; priorities are changing all around us. Although our life-style is now subdued, our joys are many and lilt of laughter is heard quite frequently in our home.

As the family plays a major role in my all-consuming fight against cancer, it seems only appropriate for me to introduce each member separately throughout this book.

I asked Bill and the children to write their own feelings, or interpretations, about how my illness had altered their lives. They were not to write about how I coped, but rather about the changes taking place in their personal lives as a result of my illness. I allowed them three months in which to submit their writing. The date was extended by three additional months since I did not receive any copy from anyone within the first three months.

Perhaps this typifies how difficult it was for them to recall unhappy times of their individual lives; perhaps the delay in responding tells me that it was too painful to explore and express their feelings. Or perhaps I am the mother of a clan of procrastinators! All completed written copy (reluctantly submitted by some, as evidenced throughout their notes and letters) was received within seven months following my request.

The family members' segments are presented in the following order: my husband, Bill, then each child in descending order, beginning with the oldest and ending with the youngest.

Bill, Sr. (My statement)

I have been blessed with an understanding husband. He helped raise the babies wholeheartedly, every bit as much a father as I am a mother. We together enjoyed the joys the family provided us and shared the sorrows we were asked to face. A single most blessing in our marriage is that Bill and I have never crumbled at the same time...when I am pessimistic about the outcome of a situation, Bill remains optimistic, and vice versa. I could never pinpoint the reason for this pattern, but recognize it as a tremendous advantage that we do not emotionally respond in a similar way under pressure. Although our "up times" are generally similarly responsive, our "down times" are not. Perhaps a bit of wisdom in recognizing when your spouse is searching for a ray of hope generates the need for a positive outlook on the part of the other.

Bill and I do not discuss my disease in detail, although I share many of my thoughts with him. Bill, in turn, keeps his own counsel. I believe he is numbed with a wrenching sorrow, looking for answers to why his wife has to endure suffering. It would be better for him, I believe, if he would express his sorrow openly. Tears need to be shed; he is allowed to grieve, to express the deep emotions within. Why do men often find it difficult to express their overwhelming sorrow?

Bill plunged willingly into the role of mother to the children in my absence, and became an apt housekeeper. This seemed to assist him in coping. Perhaps he tries to close his mind to the situation as it now exists, reluctantly accepting the fact that our lives are changed. By conscious choice, he became my protector. I am concerned how long he can console the child or children who need reassurance, work at his job daily, and assume the duties in the home that I had previously performed.

He seems distraught when I have to face something new. Questioning somewhat the drugs that cause me pain, he will not interfere with my judgement about my treatments; as long as I am positive, he'll back me up. Bill tries to spare me possibly more than I should be spared; he prefers that I perform less and take more frequent rest periods.

When throughout these two years we had to cancel many special social engagements because of side effects from chemotherapy drugs or frequent hospitalizations, Bill could accept this with me.

We openly still talk of the future looking forward to growing older together. While we were raising our family, a great deal of sacrifice was needed, including the sacrifice of time for ourselves. But the family grows, diminishes, and have their own families, and we look forward to time together again, a renewal time of our lives.

We do not refer to what we will do *next year* or the *following year*. I suppose the lack of immediate future plans is a testimonial to the awesomeness of this disease and neither of us can admit to the other that there looms some doubt. We've been a little silent in that department, and I hope it is a mutual understanding that these few years are my fighting years and "get better years." My love for Bill has only deepened with the growing dependency on him.

From Bill, Sr.:

I have started this "epistle" many times but ended up throwing it away. It just didn't seem to say what I intended. But now since all the family has written their impressions, I don't have an excuse to put it off any longer.

(Bill initially refused my request for input, stating, "it was too painful to recall." As childrens' copy arrived staggeringly, he surprised me with his input left in letter form on the pillow of my bed.)

The summer nights at home by myself gave me a chance to reflect on your battle with cancer. After reviewing our life since your first operation, I remember experiencing the following emotions (not necessarily in order).

Fear—For your health and life; for the family and myself (how could we carry on without you); for the chemo and your trips to the hospital: What did it all mean? Why so many side effects? Would the chemo help?

Outrage—Why did this have to happen to you, after a life of real giving? I still haven't gotten over this emotion, even though you seem well on your way to recovery.

Sorrow—One of the most painful experiences I had was to see you losing weight and being debilitated by the chemo. From your usual exuberant, happy, outgoing self, I could see you moving slower and slower, becoming a little thinner and not enjoying life the way you should. I didn't care that our life was more restricted, I just felt so badly that this was your reward for the years spent devoting yourself to your family.

Joy—When the surgeon told us last November that there weren't any live cancer cells visible. It was like someone lifted a ton of bricks off my shoulders. However, my joy wasn't for myself, but rather for you, that all the suffering, anxiety, sickness, etc. that you were forced to endure was finally paying off.

There were some times which were most agonizing for me. I'm not telling you about these because I was so brave (because I wasn't) but maybe you can use this in your book.

1) When the surgeon told me you had cancer. He tried not to sound pessimistic, but I felt absolutely helpless.

2) When I had to tell you that you had cancer. I didn't sleep for a couple of nights—it was hard for me but nothing like you hearing about it yourself.

3) Taking you to chemo the first time—knowing what it meant.

4) Taking you back to the hospital for platinum treatments ("Don't come to see me for a couple of days—I'll be too sick."). You must have been so lonely.

5) Calling the "Munchers" (a group of friends) after your first operation. There just wasn't any way I could talk about it.

6) Trying to comfort the kids during the first year and a half—it just seemed like your progress was at a standstill.

As I look back on that early period, it seemed so hopeless, so useless, that I wonder how we all survived.

On the other hand, there were some positive things that occurred.

1) In some small way, I was able to repay you for all the love you have given me in our past life. Taking care of you and doing for you helped me to feel as if I was helping you to get better.

2) Again, as in the many other crises we have experienced together, your determination, spunk, and zest for life won out. Without your tremendous determination and encouragement to all of us, we could not have survived. You set the tone for all of us to follow that morning at Chestnut Hill when I told you you had cancer. Your first reaction was, "I'm going to beat it! I just won't have it."

To see a person that you love so much undergo so much distress and pain was for me the hardest thing to bear during your illness and recovery. I know I became withdrawn—but I just found it very hard to talk about. I'm sure you realize I was scared to death that I would lose you. I think it's going to take quite a while before I get over it.

Something else I'm sure you noticed—I received little or no comfort from my religion or church and at the same time you found Padre Pio and renewed your devotion to the Sacred Heart. My feelings were, "Why, Kay?" Didn't she have enough suffering for one person? For me, church and religion will never be the same. I'll still go through the motions, but I don't think I can ever forgive God for the suffering he put you through.

Enough of the past. On to the future.

All I can say is that I'm so damn lucky. It seems to me that we are just on the threshold of one of the best periods in our lives. After thirty-one years, we now have time to enjoy each other. I hope you are anticipating our lives together as much as I am.

Bill, Jr. (My statement)

The oldest child in the family is our son, Bill, who is 27 years of age. He now lives in New Orleans, but was born and raised in Pennsylvania, where we reside. I must say that such a geographically distant son remains in close contact with all family members. He calls home frequently, and now with my illness, his calls average three times a week.

Bill is frightened, I suspect, about my illness and recovery. It must be difficult for him due to the fact he is such a distance, coping alone away from brother and sisters' ability to counsel one another. I anticipate that being away from the group he visualizes traumas that are not here.

When we chat on the phone together, there is a hesitation in his voice, as he remarks, "Mom, you sound tired," and I may well be exhausted just then. But the exhaustion is often temporary and I regret we probably will not be speaking together again later in the same day when Bill could hear my voice without the tiredness; but the image conjured up of my frailty will remain with him until we talk together again.

And yet he's removed from the daily complexities of chemotherapy's side effects, changes in appearance, and the decreased energy level that the other family members see as constant reminders of illness. He visits home approximately every three months, and soon experiences disappointment accompanying my illness.

Perhaps he has come to know that expressing one's anxiety feelings is a cleansing experience, natural, and should be allowed. I am not convinced he allows grief its proper necessary outlet. Bill is pensive about my illness, inclined to affect a light approach rather than reveal his inner feelings or anxiety. He is worried, I know, and yet will not allow himself tears, at least not in my presence. So I shall never know what his lonely and difficult moments are.

Bill is gifted with a spontaneous humor and makes me laugh readily, and no one enjoys a laugh better than I. Bill is a bright side of my life and an unspoken rule I detected in his youth tells me he does not like to discuss illnesses in detail, and never, but never, would bring up the subject of poor health. Bill is philosophical, and will handle my sickness his way.

From Bill I take COURAGE.

From Bill, Jr.:

This has been a difficult task to begin. The memories are painful, and recalling them, categorizing them, and committing them to an indelible state is frightening.

I remember being told of the possibilities of my mother's cancer. (Family members do not recall expressing fear of cancer or mentioning the word cancer to Bill or each other. Bill recalls during our phone conversation the night before surgery that I said "they'll check me during surgery to make sure I don't have 'The Big C'.") *This recollection is vague, however. It is overshadowed by the poignant announcement that shocked us all.*

I was in Baton Rouge on the day of the exploratory operation. My colleague and I were presenting a seminar. The preparations for the seminar helped take my mind off the operation and the consequences of the findings. When I called the family from the hotel in Baton Rouge and heard my father's voice, I realized for the first time that my mother's life had an end. As a son, I knew little of my mother's beginnings—who would? She was always there from the first of my memories through the present. Why shouldn't she always be there? The picture of a finality had not occurred to me. The novelty of that thought helped lessen the pain. Why had I been so unaware? I marveled at the isolation of the concept. We had been so close for my whole life. Had she lived her life as fully as she had hoped?

The ride from Baton Rouge to New Orleans was very long. I was with a business colleague who owed me no emotional support. I told him the news, of course, but I couldn't share my anguish. Even in New Orleans, I quickly learned not to share my grief. Cancer is an evil disease in the minds of most people. They just don't want to talk about it. I can't blame them, and I won't attempt to find comfort in others anymore. I have learned that my strength is inside me. I'm glad to know that; it saves time.

My father told me on the phone that it was a shame that I didn't have the rest of the family around to help me through this time. My brother told me that they needed my strength; I'm sorry I wasn't home to give of myself, but I'm glad I didn't have to live with all these sad people. I would have, but it was easier to be alone.

I never really believed that my mother would survive her cancer until this summer (1982). I worked overtime to finish my doctoral program so my mother could live to see me receive my Ph.D. This is not to say that all my intentions in this area were selfless. Previously, I wanted to stop being a student. Secondarily, while I did want my mother at the ceremony, it was so that she would be proud of me. That this is a selfish deed is plain to me. It is also the most painful aspect of my memories. I not only wanted my mother to live for her own sake, but also for my own edification. When a close friend pointed this out in an accusatory manner, my guilt was, and still is, crushing.

While I was taking classes for my Ph.D. two years ago, I wrote letters to myself in the margins of my class notes. I knew I'd be reviewing my notes this past year. The message was short for the class after my trip to Baton Rouge.

"Just found out that Mom has cancer." It hurt to re-read it.

My mother survived. She paid a heavy price, but is there a price that is too high? I don't believe there is. I love her no more now than I did before, but I am surely aware of her as a person, as a being. I've learned a great deal about sharing joy and grief. I know now that I can live with grief. I've learned not to spread it around or try to share it. It has its place in our lives. Without it, joy would be meaningless. I still don't look upon it in a spiritual sense. That is for others perhaps, but not for me. I'm close to my family because I know that I have an impact upon them. Yet in a way, I'm more distant also, because I know that in the end, we are all alone.

Diane (My statement)

The second oldest child is our daughter, Diane, age 26. Diane is perhaps, I would venture to say, taking this illness the most openly and with great difficulty. She understands in part the treatments I must endure, the endless amount of blood work performed, the weekly intramuscular and intravenous probing of needles, the discomfort caused by collapsed veins no longer able to accommodate a needle.

Diane is a diabetic and presents first hand knowledge of what accompanies a prolonged, chronic disease. She handles her own health problems quite well but appears to have difficulty in accepting mine. Also, it strikes me that Diane is resistant to my withdrawal into meditation. She once expressed her feelings quite well in saying, "I feel as though there are times I cannot seem to reach you."

She has the ability to strip away the outer veneer covering my emotions, perhaps probing for the truth of my acceptance of this battle. This inward searching stems from her knowledge of medicine and procedures, gained when she worked as a medical technician and doctor's assistant in hospitals. Diane has seen the ravage of cancer a little too closely. I truly believe she is riddled with doubts about a complete recovery for me, a role reversal that I am most unhappy with. It is my wish she not suffer for me.

Many times throughout her early teens and twenties, her Dad and I sat beside her hospital bed thinking we were going to lose her to diabetes, and I thank God he has not asked us to accept what I believe to be the ultimate sacrifice of losing a child in death.

Diane and I both recognize she needs my support in grave situations and now the only supportive role I can assume is a positive attitude that eventually I am to be rid of cancer.

She has, I know, a fear in her that I will not make it, unspoken but there.

Diane and her husband, Fred, are the parents of a daughter, Nicole. This interruption in her young married years must be a drain on her, as she comes to her parents' home almost daily to help with the care I sometimes need.

From Diane I take DEVOTION.

From Diane:

The most important thing I have learned from this whole experience is how to help a person live with cancer. As a medical assistant to various doctors for the past eight years, I have learned to accept the deaths of many patients. I have learned how not to get too involved, too concerned, too emotional and how to help them accept their own deaths. But my mother has brought a whole new meaning to the word "cancer" for me. I will no longer associate an original diagnosis of cancer with the word "death." I now think of it as being simultaneous with "fight." It is certainly a long road with many peaks and valleys along the way, but with the encouragement of family and friends and a sheer desire to live, a cancer patient may very well become one of those who "make it."

Looking back to the very beginning, I find myself very critical of the medical profession in general. Why did they never mention the word "cancer" to us during the days prior to my mother's surgery when performing various tests. I am angry with myself for not preparing my family for the news. Surely the doctors must have suspected but they never let on to us that there might be a malignancy. Why couldn't someone have sat down with us and said, "We think everything will be fine, but you should be prepared, just in case, that your wife/mother may possibly have cancer." Would that have lessened the blow? I really couldn't say for sure, but I think getting it out in the open would have made it somewhat easier for the diagnosis that was to follow. I often thought of it during the days prior to her surgery, but I thought since "they" didn't talk about it that I must be overreacting. And why expose my family to my groundless fears?—or so we thought. What about the days to follow in the hospital? I have often helped attend men and women in the first few days after a major heart attack in the Intensive Care Unit of the hospital. During their first critical days, they had no more of a chance of recovering from a major heart attack than my Mom did, at the time, of recovering from cancer. Indeed, their chance of death was greater at the time than that of my mother's but the difference in care was astounding. Why does the cancer patient have to deal with the medical profession's avoidance of eye contact, the doctors and nurses who are afraid to touch them, to reach out and put a hand on their shoulder for reassurance, or merely to sit beside them on their bed rather than stand stiffly at the end of it? Surely, there were exceptions, but they were certainly in the minority. One does get the feeling that there isn't much hope and yet the patient hasn't ever received a first treatment which could begin to bring about a recovery!

There were many times when I didn't think she would make it. During her platinum therapy, I knew that approximately one hour after the I.V. was completed she would have tremendous bouts of nausea and vomiting and that it would last for approximately twenty-four hours. I could seldom sleep those nights thinking of what she was going through. I rejoiced in my heart when I knew she would be sleeping from exhaustion and another treatment would be completed. We all shared in her happiness when those hospital trips were over, but knew they were necessary as one of the major factors in her recovery.

During those times, my father, brothers, sisters and myself spent hours on the phone supporting each other.

To those of you reading this book, I wish you hope. You would not read this book if you didn't have a close family member or friend with cancer. Hopefully, you are reading this book in the early stages of their treatment. It will not be easy. You will suffer right along with the cancer patient. Your heart will break when you see them changed from the way you always knew them. If you believe in a Supreme Being, you will pray harder than you ever have before to have this patient's life spared. Perhaps like myself, your reasons may even be slightly selfish ones. You want this person's life spared, yes, for herself and the joys that lie ahead for her; but also for yourself, because you need her and because you couldn't imagine life without her.

So many wonderful things lie ahead for my family and for myself, and I'm so happy that my mom will be here to share them with us—for she is one of those who "made it."

John (My statement)

Our third child is a son, John, who is 25. He is analytical and I feel strengthened in that I believe he expects me completely to recover, given time. John asks about the treatment received, the possible side effects, and my reactions. He listens and in some instances does not feel I should accept drugs without knowing the possible side effects. He feels some radical treatments are an "overkill" and is not convinced I am in need of certain drugs. However, he has an earthy realization of the magnitude of the battle I am fighting and acquiesces in my judgment. When I speak of the anticipation within me of a miracle, John's reply is, "Mother, sometimes miracles happen and sometimes people make them happen." This remark speaks of both his strength and mine, and many times I've recalled this statement as a source of reinforcement. He sees me as having a bright, optimistic outlook and does not appear to have any doubts about my living. Nor do I feel he questions "WHY" this disease has reared its ugly presence. This realism is shared by John and me, as through the years I have stopped asking "WHY." Answers are not directly forthcoming and the searching for explanations weighs heavily where there is no answer. John shares his anguish openly, but grieves privately. Tenderness is ever present as extended hands grasp mine and the subject is faced squarely between mother and son, and silent tears are shed. John remains at home, at his suggestion, for the durations of my illness. Therefore we meet every day. John does not attempt to escape from life's happenings and offers solace.

From John I take STRENGTH.

From John:

How was I affected by my mother's bout with cancer? A question which no one wishes to have the experience to answer.

Nevertheless, the circumstances occurred, and I was consequently affected. The effect on me, and I dare to say on all members of the family, was somewhat tempered by my mother's ability to confront her disease with self assurance and emotional stability. I was aware that my mother possessed these attributes, but not to the extent to which they were tested. She unquestionably eased the emotional burden on all of us by her undying self-determination to live.

I never understood what cancer was, how it affected people, least of all how it affected cancer patients' families and friends. I had an acquaintance in college who died shortly after graduation from cancer. I don't remember at this time what kind of cancer it was, but I remember seeing him without his hair, and he took on disproportionate characteristics, in terms of being one time very thin and another time being very puffy, and I recall my heart going out to him sympathetically for the fact that he had to go through this terrible pain and suffering, and relief, I think, when I heard that he died—at least his suffering was over. In terms of cancer affecting our family personally, I never really thought that would happen, just like you never think you'll be the one mugged, be in a car accident, be the one affected by any catastrophic disease, and yet it happened.

I helped Dad make phone calls that night (of surgery) to dear friends; one friend in particular said that the news was very bad, that very few people ever recovered from ovarian cancer. I didn't know anything about it at that time and did not realize the odds were that bad. I remember thinking my mother could be a fugitive from the law of statistics, as I heard it said once before about a cancer patient who lived in the face of all odds. I called a friend from law school, and he was the opposite—ridiculously optimistic that everything would be all right, trying to give reassurance. And I remember saying to him, "We have to be realistic. My mother may die. But I'm not going to be accepting of a predetermination of that outcome."

I think the worst thing about trying to deal with catastrophic illness is that you allow it to consume you, and you can no longer be a productive person. You become absorbed in one thing and it unbalances your entire life and I knew that if anyone would not want that, it would be my mother, and I knew that the temptation was truly there and yet we all had to go on.

If I could offer some suggestions to those who might read this book, I think the first suggestion I would make is that the cancer patient himself needs the most help. If the patient sees others dealing with the situation in a positive fashion, I think it helps him deal with it as well.

Secondly, I think trying to solve and deal with the problem alone is not only difficult, I think it is foolish. You've got to reach out and touch and be touched by other persons whether they be family members or not. The family is easier to lean on, but I do not think it necessarily has to be that way.

The third point is that you must always be realistic with regard to what is happening. Be super sensitive to the feelings of others, but don't be so positive in your attitude that you begin to believe nothing is wrong or it's all going to be all right because many of you who read this book will not be as fortunate as I and will lose your loved one. I think it is important to be prepared for that. I know I was, as much as one can be while the person is still alive.

The fourth point would be that you've got to rely very strongly on the medical profession. Even though they are inflicting a lot of pain and suffering, it's at this point a necessity. The perspective you need to maintain is that the pain and suffering is purposeful; it is leading to the ultimate goal. It's a common saying amongst the military, I have heard, that you've got to lose some battles to win the war. The war in this instance is against cancer; the victory is life. Battles which you lose are physical comfort, the freedom from pain. From the perspective of a family member, I think it is important to remember that you are fighting more than the disease itself; you are fighting emotional stress; you are fighting a psychological impediment.

You must carry on; you've got to proceed in your own individual life and help others to do the same. To be absorbed with the last days, if it's that close, or the years of treatment as in the case of my mother, to be totally absorbed with that problem or to be totally absorbed with the ramifications of that problem provides no benefit to anyone, least of all the cancer patient. It seems to me that my mother was watching very carefully how each of us would live without her in the event she should die, how we would go on. I suspect very strongly she had in her mind a checklist she was going to go down in her last couple of days and say this is what I see as the weakness of one and the strengths of another, and you've all got to pull together. I think it is important you leave a cancer patient, at whatever stage, with the feeling that his/her family will continue to go on and survive and will aid in helping each other with the situation after death as well as during life. I really felt that my mother was watching that, and it was important for me that we leave her with some sort of reassurance that we would be very helpful to one another. I thank God every night we weren't faced with that problem.

I encourage you to pray for there is much comfort in putting things in someone else's hands and relieving yourself of the burden by saying, "God, I put it in your hands; your will be done." I got a tremendous amount of comfort from doing that.

Those of you that read this book out of curiosity rather than being affected, I encourage you to pray as well that you will never have to bear the burden that one bears in a situation like this. I wish I could say I am better off for it, but I can't—I would have been better off without it.

Maliz (My statement)

Maliz is our fourth child, 24 years of age. She and her husband, Lou, drove five hours the night of my surgery to bring a sister, Cindy, home from college. Maliz is gentle. I can only envision the hugging, flow of tears, and exchange of questions that took place when these two sisters embraced each other with a shared sorrow. Maliz' eyes are both large and expressive. We, mother and daughter, can look into each other's eyes, not speak a word, and recognize each other's feelings. It is easy for me to realize the compassion offered behind the tears she holds back. Sometimes escaped tears moisten her cheeks and glide downward beguiling the serenity of her expression as doubt creeps into her mind about my health, her rational thinking sustaining her.

However, I think Maliz believes so strongly in what I believe that she is convinced I will be cured, reinforcing my thoughts with her belief.

Maliz frequently comes home after her day's work to visit the family. We talk intimately, and her ability to put priorities in perspective helps me, as she, the loving observer, brings the gift of serenity.

Maliz has the beautiful capacity to stand silently at my bedside and transfer her love with a spiritual depth.

From Maliz I take COMPASSION.

From Maliz:

Before your book is released into its tenth printing, I thought I'd better write this for you!

It was difficult for me to put into words the feeling I had two years ago. Not because I have forgotten how I felt (which I haven't) but because I felt overwhelmed when your illness was diagnosed as cancer.

A few experiences I had still are very clear to me. First, I really surprised myself with how I reacted to the news. Up until then, I sort of though of myself as someone who comforts or could keep up with confidence when things were not going well. But when I heard what the surgeon said after the operation, I really grieved. I couldn't find it within myself to try to comfort the other family members because I couldn't reassure myself. People would tell me that they knew someone who had had the same type of cancer and who was doing fine after treatment. But it didn't matter to me who had what; this was my mother; it was different. I think it was because I allowed myself this time to sort out my feelings that I was able to be myself more easily than if I had tried to ignore or suppress my feelings. Instead, I acknowledged that it was okay to be angry at the unfairness of it all, and it helped me react a little better.

You know, Mom, it's really a great network of family of which we are a part. I drew on family members for comfort and support and others came to me for help. It seemed that when one person felt the hurt and uncertainty overwhelming, there was always someone else who was able to see something positive to reassure them. If I had a day of worry and spoke of this to Lou, his mood was encouraging, warm and calming. Or on another day, he might voice his concern to me and I was able to help and reassure him. All involved—husbands, Dad, sisters and brothers—each played a role in helping the others over the rough times. And for that, I'm sure we are all thankful.

But most of all, Mom, it was you who helped us all keep going. Imagine, we all had our energies concentrating on your health and well being, but you had all of us to concern yourself with!

I still marvel at your spirit and unwavering faith and confidence. You have shown us a valuable lesson in the meaning of giving and sharing in life and that life is for living every day.

Joan (My statement)

Our next child, our fifth, is our daughter, Joan, who is 22 years of age. Joan lives totally apart from the family by her choice. She knows I am a cancer patient.

Joan is not aware of the trials the family shares, nor does she address the existence of my illness when we are in contact. She must face life in her own fashion. That is the type of person she has been from late teens onward.

In the exchange of letters between us, I have sent medals of Padre Pio, hoping the extension of his love will shower her with the warmth and desire to be closer to her sisters and brothers, and perhaps even close to her parents.

I hope there will be a day when Joan is in more frequent contact with us, more a part of the family than the previous years have brought.

From Joan I take HOPE.

Cindy (My statement)

The unruffled, calm expression of Cindy's face seemingly expresses an inner peace. I particularly recall times of her childhood when while the family gathered at the dinner table in all the confusion seven children can create, Cindy sat calmly like a Hummel figurine of a child, peace of soul evident through her composure, always renewing tranquility in me. Cindy is now 19 years old and continues to be blessed with a complacency that assures me she has met with life and has chosen to keep anxiety at a distance.

During my illness and while holding my hand, she would inquire about my condition, and yet I recognized a hesitancy in her, not wanting to hear in depth about illness, because although she wants to be physically near, I know in reality she will not want to share fears that accompany illness, rather choosing to confide her concerns with her older sisters and privately coping with her anxieties, preferring to withhold her uncertainty from me. I do feel that she, too, is doubtful my confidence in a complete recovery is justified.

We have walked arm in arm, at my slowed pace, across her college campus with her concern for my fragility worn as a badge before her peers, she stronger than I physically, and seemingly more peaceful than I.

Her composure was betrayed a few times during phone calls to me when I was hospitalized, when she cried while seeking reassurance that I would be okay. Perhaps in her mind we are both more vulnerable while she is away from the family at school, and I am away from the family in the hospital.

From Cindy I take PEACE.

From Cindy:

There is no question that my family and friends were the reason for my being able to cope with and accept my mother's illness. Support, encouragement and above all, love were always in abundance for me.

I always tried hard to be strong for my family. This is part of my nature, and I felt that it was my most important contribution at the time. It was comforting to know that they needed me as much as I needed them. I felt as though no matter what happened, we would get through it, together.

Being away at college during my mother's illness made it very difficult for me at times. But my loneliness and fear were soothed by a hug or a reassuring word from a good friend. Each person expressed concern and love in a unique and special way. This meant the world to me then and now.

My father, my sisters and brothers, and my friends gave so much to me the past two years. But the person I counted on most was my mother her-

self. I knew from the moment she said she would beat the cancer that she would live. Among other things, I greatly appreciated her encouragement to continue on with our lives as they were before. Cancer, chemotherapy, platinum treatments, etc. become part of my life, and I learned to accept them as such.

There are many feelings and emotions that occurred during the last couple of years that I simply cannot write about. At times, I have shared these thoughts with someone very close to me, and at other times, I have kept them to myself. Because for me, it didn't matter whether I spoke my feelings or kept them inside; I knew those who were close to me understood.

Jeannine (My statement)

Our seventh and youngest child is Jeannine, age 15. She is a worrier and a doer. Jeannine willingly assumed my previous chores around the home, wanting to help in whatever capacity needed.

Such a giving child, willing to run a myriad of errands that couldn't be completed in one day. I look at Jeannine and pray, please Lord, don't let her develop the hurried pace I had allowed myself to develop. Let her know peace of mind and slower steps.

I feel my illness is extremely hard for her. She, too, is at home each day and spends a great deal of time talking with me about her concerns. Her face readily reveals her anxiety and I weep secretly that my illness is depriving Jeannine of some of her childhood years.

The day following surgery, I told Jeannine, "I'll dance at your wedding," and I feel she expects me to have restored health but in watching me do daily battle with chemo side effects, she suffers intently. We share both laughter and sorrow together. Jeannine is a grown child now; adversity shoved childhood play aside and a wondrous, warm, understanding woman emerged ready to aid her family in time of turmoil, and with insurmountable willingness.

We share thoughts of happy times and confide in one another our love, she maintaining an air of capability, and I comforted by her youthful understanding of life's adversities.

From Jeannine I take JOY.

From Jeannine:

I had asked my dad to come pick me up at school and take me down to the hospital to be with two of my sisters and him while they waited to hear the outcome of Mom's operation. To this day, I'm grateful Dad came to get me because as soon as we arrived at the hospital, we were to hear, together, the terrible news from my sisters and experience the shock they had been given. When we walked into the doctor's office, I saw that the girls had been crying. I thought maybe Mom had died, but I couldn't find the courage to ask. My sister Diane told us that they had found a lump and it was malignant, we all began to cry. I wasn't even sure at the time what "malignant" meant. When it occurred to me that Mom might not live long, I thought first of the little things we did together, like shopping, kidding each other, joking, and just lying across her bed and talking. My first thoughts not only revolved around how much I was going to miss my mother, but also how much I was going to miss my very good friend.

The night of Mom's operation, I came to realize just how much my family meant to me. We were always close, but that night we had to lean and depend on each other like never before. If I needed help, there was always somebody right there beside me offering advice or comforting words. If no words could be found, they simply lent their shoulder for me to cry

*on. This pattern has continued right up until this day, and I believe it al-
ways will. I think this is what helped me most, knowing that members of the
family were always there if I needed them. I think we all felt compelled to
look out for each other. I remember thinking that first night, "I'm the only
girl at home now, and I'm gonna have to look after Dad and take care of
Mom. I have to be brave. The family has enough to worry about without
worrying about me." Yet it seemed that over the difficult times it was my
dad who looked out for me, and my brothers and sisters were the first ones
I ran to when I when I needed help. For me, it was easy to think such
thoughts but much harder to carry them out.*

*Throughout these past two years, I have relied heavily on my family,
and I drew something from each member, whether it was advice, reassurance, comfort, strength and even laughter.*

*I think my position in the family changed, too. Suddenly I was no longer
the baby. My family never tried to hide anything from me, and for that I
will always be grateful. Since Mom's diagnosis of cancer, I feel I have
been treated as an adult and everyone has talked and listened to me as an
adult. Although I feel I have grown up a lot within these past two years, I
don't feel as if I have missed out on my childhood. Mom's illness rarely
prevented me from going out with my friends and enjoying the time spent
with them. I've found some welcome relief with them when things were
tough at home.*

*I think I have become closer to Mom since her diagnosis of cancer. We
have been able to spend more time together, and I feel I know her even better than I did before her illness. Since Mom has become sick, she sometimes needs my help and it makes me feel good to be able to help her instead of Mom always helping me. I want to listen to her and hear what the
doctors are going to do to help cure her. As I look back now, I can see how
strange it is that I knew and cared so little about a disease and within
hours, it can become the most important thing in my life. Up until Mom's
diagnosis, I thought that cancer was just cancer—there were no specific
kinds, and I thought there were no treatments except radiation. I only knew
that radiation was painful, and it made me hurt to think of what I thought*

Mom would have to go through. Over the years, I feel I have become very informed on cancer, and sometimes I knew more that I think I cared to know. I had read a little about cancer and the statistics of people who survived, and I knew only too well that cancer was something to be feared. In the months following Mom's diagnosis, I feared it a lot. Today, though, I don't fear it very much. Cancer can still give me a scare, but I guess I have grown used to it because it has become part of my life, and it's a part of reality—something I realize must be faced and met head on. I know now cancer is sometimes possible to overcome and that Mom will conquer it.

11.
The Clergy: Their Pastoral Role

I'll remember you
at the altar of God.

Rev. John J. Fitzpatrick, S. J.

During repeated hospitalizations over a period of 22 months, I grew as a thinker. I had time to observe. Time is a curious commodity. When we are told we might not have much of it, it seems to be all that we have. Another paradox.

One observation is this: if dying is the business of the soul, then so must be living. When was it I heard "There are no agnostics on the battlefield?" I cannot remember who said it but it's true. The battlefield here from my hospital bed is death from cancer. I observe others in the dying process, there are no agnostics here. We have souls. The soul is a sacred place. Our sacredness. The location is illusive. Is it the organs? The heart? The glands? Or is it our consciousness?

85

Can humans talk soul to soul? We do communicate heart to heart in love. But soul to soul; can that be done? If so, then by whom?

Is my expectation of clergy unrealistic if I expect that their counsel will bring peace to my soul? Is that type of searching possible with the ordained of the Church? A rabbi? A minister? A priest?

My observations were that some clergy engage and console. Some never get past the magic wall at the foot of the bed. Some are better, in my view, at what they set out to do than others. What then is 'my view'? It is this: We are people, fellow human beings, frail, easily shattered and alone in this world. No one is more alone than when they face death or the prospect of an extended illness. Health ambulates us. Propels us through this world. When we lose it we understand, painfully so, how very tenuous our hold on this life can be. For those of us who believe in God, or simply believe in a Higher Power, or a place more vast and deeper then this, we need validation that someone cares about our souls. To say that we are not alone is not true. We are. Our acknowledgement of that experiential reality is what makes congregation so sweet. We gather at a place to hold hands, to break bread, to share the Eucharist. We acknowledge essential aloneness *en masse*. Perhaps the congregation is our crucible, our validation, our salvation.

What, then, is a clergy supposed to represent in the role of comforter/comforting? Is the definition clear in what they are trained to be, and what the layman expects them to be? Or are the translations different? Are all ordained ministers truly adequate in reaching out to the very sick and the dying? Of course not. They, like you and I, are people. We vary do we not? What then do we want from these men and women of the cloth? I believe we want a symbol; a link between us and our God. Dying is a business of the soul. It is deep, moving and inexact. It is fraught with worry, doubt and fear. We need a symbol that congeals all that. Allows it form. Severe illness draws much the same responses from us. We who are ill understand the link between the spirit and the body. We have felt how difficult it can be to maintain spiritual health when our bodies have shaken us at our foundations. For these things we need our clergy. I think too that we need to see them as people.

Often, as I lay in bed and consider my plight, I wonder about the spiritual well-being of my family. You already know of Bill's experience. My opinion is that God can deal with our anger at Him. It disappoints me knowing that at no time did my family receive pastoral care. They would have benefitted from that. I hope the clergy will embrace this singular mission. Teach it to their students. Cancer is a family affair. My family would have been uplifted by a direct "and how are you doing" and caring about their response. The ordained proclamation that somebody cared about the soul of them.

I have heard fellow patients mention the moment of spiritual well-being felt when clergy entered their hospital room. This may be temporary but it forms a frame of reference; a time when we felt okay about who we were and the situation in which we found ourselves.

An interesting observation is that just as visitors come in twos; most clergy come alone. Hence, what they say is heard, calculated and reminisced. I wanted to believe they understood: God did not send me a cross because I am strong. My strength is not superhuman. Nor does God try most those he loves the best. God does not love me the best, nothing about His love for me or mine is measured. I want the clergy to assure me they understand LIFE is illuminated more beautifully as it flickers. Help me with that.

Just as I admired the physician who called the specialist when he felt in-adequate to help me...so do I admire the clergy who did not assume to have all the answers and said, "I'll pray for you." He too called upon the specialist.

Maybe that should be our expectation of these men and women. Simple caring. Simple sharing.

12.
Friends

Friends,
I pray that I am as much for you
as you are for me.
My friend, I love you.

Diane Westlake

Let the soul be assured that somewhere in the universe it should
rejoin its friend, and it would be content and cheerful alone for a
thousand years.

—Ralph Waldo Emerson

Friendship and all that it brings to us plays a major role in life and
recovery. I have no doubt that friends make life worth living and I have
been blessed by both the number and the variety of my friends.

Visitors generally came in twos and threes to the hospital. It was a comfort knowing that my closest friends were not afraid and came as soon as
they could or as soon as they knew. In the months that followed I had
deeply personal encounters where my condition and all the myriad possibilities were openly discussed. I did not feel awkward in these discussions, but validated. I was cared for by another human being. So simple,
and yet what courage I took from them.

89

Friends, and these encounters, brought the world to me. Made me want to get going again. Resume my life and feel the sun in my face. That kind of feeling is what they brought with them to my side and sometimes I wondered how one lived without these people. I loved and love them still, and they love me. I've no doubt of that.

Notes and letters sent from my friends would fill volumes. Their words were words of hope, of love and sincerity. Their wishes for me were of health and recovery. For my family their wishes were for courage and strength and good spirits. Their love took the shape of meals and desserts and to this day I have not returned all the casserole dishes nor will I ever find who owns them all.

Many of the words of my friends are indelible. They shall not leave me ever. I'll share a few with you.

"What I read in your letter was an earned peace of the soul, a vivid faith, an earthy acceptance of reality—and a light-heartedness that can come only from inside, from meeting what's real and being creative with it. And take credit, you needn't at all have gone that route. You chose to. The Lord is greatly in it all; but you had to want Him there." Father G.

"Just finished talking with you on the phone, and I have been uplifted. Thought it was going to be the other way around." B.M.

"You have given me many lessons of love and courage and joy, and I know that you will give me many more. I hope I can in some way return your gift with my love and courage and joy." M.H.

"I hope Padre Pio's intercession to the Lord will bring about a cure. Faith is the thing!" Fr. F.

"What words of wisdom can I write for you—keep your wonderful zest for living and your faith. Have you asked God to knock it off lately?" M.B.

"For continued improvement." M.L.

A lifelong friend of mine, a priest, sent me a news clipping. The story told was of a conversation between Mother Teresa of Calcutta and a young college girl, dying of terminal cancer. "Pray to be weak," Mother Teresa, a living saint, had told the girl. It is not easy for us to accept weakness, but in this condition God works His Will through us. "In strength, we try to direct our lives, but in weakness, we let the Lord do the directing."

I had nurtured just the opposite approach. I want to share a prayer with you. It is called the Serenity Prayer: "God grant me the Serenity to accept the things I cannot change; Courage to change the things I can, and Wisdom to know the difference."

It took me a long time to understand the meaning in my friend's news clipping. We fight our situations. We resist the situations in which we find ourselves for a mountain of "right" reasons. But we invest so much energy into this resistance that we lose touch with our need to accept. Yes, I need to be strong to fight this disease but I do not have to spend energy on wishing that my situation were otherwise. I must depend upon my family and my friends now. That is my situation. I can accept that "weakness" and find comfort in that. An unplanned truce. My separate peace.

I did not now think of "weak" as a permanent condition, but, rather, as a vantage from which to begin my fight. I will become stronger. I know God wants me to live. Life and friendship are interchanged now. Friends truly bring life to my door. They make life impose upon me. Yet the imposition is not negative. Their concern keeps life railing at my door and if we can interchange Life and God, then the gift these people, these friends bring to me is finest gift of all.

A friend from high school days called. "We're having dinner Kay. At your house." I picked a date from four options. My friend and her husband arrived at 5:30 with everything from hors d'oeuvres to dessert. They even brought the coffeepot, complete with electric cord and coffee. Dinner was served an hour later and they left at half past eight. That was living! I was alive and my friend brought that realization home to Bill and I in our home in a very direct way. I love them.

I have laughed with my friends over wearing my wig. I have opened my door to boxes of candy and well wishing cards. Flowers from the gardens of those I love have watched with me in hospital rooms and one Easter morning a friend stopped by on her way home from church. "I just wanted to drop this plant off to you before breakfast," she said. She stood in my home in Easter frills and fought back tears at my appearance. She understood what her visit meant to me. I had just returned home from my last cis-platinum treatment. I needed the lift and her visit, again, brought life reeling back to me.

Friends will do all they can in their varied ways to let you know that life awaits you. Some will let you know that someone else is worse off than you. Others will hold "hen" parties with and for you. Some will talk of anything but your illness and still others will engage you and allow you to share thoughts that, perhaps, you haven't even verbalized to yourself. It is all so very needed. I've got some advice to share for anyone who wants to know the protocols of caring. Here goes:

My experience is that spontaneous, unannounced visits to a hospitalized patient are welcomed during visiting hours. However, if a patient is pre-operative he/she is often out of the room having tests in the daytime. This is especially so in large teaching hospitals. Generally, community hospitals leave the visiting hours free.

In cases of severe illness, or powerful chemotherapy treatments, it is better not to visit. Just call the family. They can advise whether or not the patient is up to visiting. The family can also relay the fact of your call.

When a patient returns home, very close friends and relatives are welcomed either announced or unannounced. Common sense dictates the best route to take.

Generally, it is more comfortable for the patient if a phone call is made or a note dropped off, asking what time of day is best for a visit. There are generally up and down times during the day.

Often friends would just drop by and ask how I was doing, and did not feel it was necessary to visit with me. My family felt comfortable enough to convey the situation to them at the time.

The best advice I can give is to make a contact with which YOU are comfortable. If you are afraid of illness and perhaps particularly afraid of seeing a person with cancer and in failing health, you can just call or write a note. It really is the thought that counts. All contacts are reinforcing.

To all my friends I must tell you: I love you. Thank you for your friendship. It means my life to me!

13.
Chemotherapy
Friends

Unchartered Paths

A common bond;
sharing fears
hiding tears

A knowing glance
looking beyond
into the heart of another.

—Kay Quain

Prologue

Chemotherapy ends. It is the slow unfolding of a promise: remission, cure!

You can see it in their eyes. Hope! Sitting in the oncologist's office week after week you cannot help but see it shining through. We are in hiatus. A limbo of waiting for the return of our health and a new life. We

95

climb over each other, figuratively. We are all growing within a paradox. While seemingly dying; we are all learning more about life than we ever imagined.

We are brothers-in-arms! Hands are stretched across this subjective battlefield. We meet. We share triumphs when one of our number is soon to complete chemotherapy. Graduation! And we share bad times too. But God how we learn; one from the other. More and more of us graduate and one of these is Lil.

I want you to meet her. Lil: a chemo friend of mine. We are as different as night is to day. Our common bond is obvious.

Lil is serene and most attractive. A beautiful 50. She wants to know as little as possible about her disease. She desires to affect an aloofness. She will make it easy for our doctor to keep his schedule. She'll ask no questions.

"I become upset when someone does not show up for weekly treatment," she says. "I fear they have died or become severely ill."

Lil does not like waiting with other patients in the doctor's office. This has made her consider changing physicians. Lil and I are nearly comlete opposites I soon realize. She needs not to know. I need every scrap of information I can gather. When a patient enters the office, sallow and sunken-eyed Lil averts her eyes. She does not want any confrontation with this disease. She shall be a bystander in her treatment.

Each chemo injection makes Lil sick to her stomach. She managed some comfort at knowing that, like her, I was bald too.

This lady has Hodgkin's Disease. Her second bout, following a remission that lasted 22 years. This is news to her. When first diagnosed her husband kept the information from her. That was her first husband who died. On a vacation with her second husband she discovered swollen lymph nodes on either side of her neck. An investigation turned up the first diagnosis. Her first husband knew that she "would not want to know."

Lil's husband's first wife died of cancer. This adds to her burden as she deals with the anxiety evident on his face.

This woman will deny that she is courageous. I disagree. She shields the burden from her parents. During visits with them they comment on her new hairstyle. She covers with a story and hopes they do not realize she is wearing a wig.

Lil's battle has had complications. Severe wretching from the chemo caused a hernia. She was hospitalized three times due to phlebitis further complicated by pneumonia. She fears hospitals greatly and feels that interns put you at risk because "they lack experience." "Cancer patients are better off in big city hospitals," she says. "Because larger hospitals are better staffed."

Lil's husband and family rally around her with the utmost support. Her chances are good she feels. Hodgkin's sometimes responds to treatments and they feel since she pulled through the first time she will again.

It amazes me that this woman is unaware of her ability to encourage others. She brings with her a radiiant healthful appearance and an endearing presence.

In preparation for this manuscript she told me that it (the interview) wasn't "as bad as I expected. I thought it was going to be a problem. It's hard for me to talk about it (cancer). I feel better now that I have. She wants "to get on with living again."

Meet another friend named Dave:

Picture him sprawled across his hospital bed; dungarees; sneakers and sport shirt. Exuding an urgency to "get going," Dave is a spunky 22 year old non-conformist, fighting testicular cancer. He has already been through nine months of weekly chemotherapy including five cis-platinum treatments. He remains resilient, determined and optimistic.

Dave's current prognosis is positive. Initially this was not so. The oncologist told Dave when he was first diagnosed that if he did not undergo a stringent chemotherapy regimen he would be dead in six months. Tough news at any age but, at 22, Dave met it with determination. He laughed when he first heard the news. "I don't know why I laughed," he adds quickly.

I met him during this chemo regimen, as he was entering the hospital for this sixth and last cis-platinum treatment. His weekly injections, though, would continue for many months, into years.

Our only obvious common bond is cancer. Nothing else. Each of us has a cancer impossible for the other. Mine of the ovaries; his of the testicles. Yet our bonds, though not obvious are very real. Both have endured six cis-platinum treatments and weekly chemotherapy. Each of us too has a deep trust in both God and our oncologist.

This man has been emotionally catapulted from youth into the worry that accompanies a life-threatening disease. He has made decisions about the course of treatment; been concerned about the expenses incurred in this battle and dealt with the lingering thoughts of death at an early age. He has literally earned extra months of life.

Our conversation was protracted. Dave, at 22, is an interesting human being with a unique perspective on this life.

After chatting briefly and informally, our conversation took on interview form. I asked questions, and Dave freely and willingly shared his responses.

Q. Dave, briefly describe to me how you reacted to hearing the news you are a cancer patient?

A. When I came to a little bit from surgery (for removal of the testicular tumor), I was surrounded by family, my parents, sister, aunts and uncles, and girlfriend. They were crying, but it didn't faze me why they were crying, I was in so much pain...the pain was overriding my emotions. When I woke the next day, I asked the nurse what the doctor had said, and she told me, "Yes, it is cancer," and the surgeon would recommend me to a good doctor. She said she had seen this cancer before and knew some people who did get better. Later the same day, it was suggested to Dave by the doctor that he go in an ambulance that night to the Health Cancer Institute in Washington for six months. "The doctor told me all costs would be paid for because this institute was interested in the exact type of cancer I had." Dave fought that idea and said he would hold off for awhile. "Things were happening just too quickly, and in the six months I would not get to come home or be with my family. I found out instead that I would be able to get good health care right in this area (Philadelphia). I was recommended to the oncologist and I felt everything started working out real good."

Q. How were you able to talk about your health problem with your friends, and what were their reactions to your disease?

A. The first couple weeks were real hard. They would stop around to see me, and one time in particular, I remember a good friend said to me, "I wanted to stop over now before you start getting real sick." He wanted to see me before I started getting thinner and sicker, but I could never see that happening to me. You don't hear about people getting cured from cancer and I think my friends didn't know that, but I always felt I would get better.

Q. How about your mother and dad, Dave? Are they able to handle your illness?

A. I had to stay strong for my parents' sake, and when I was being strong, they were strong too. But like today (when Dave entered the hospital for the sixth cis-platinum treatment) it's really hard on my parents. They're working and yet they feel they should be here at the hospital, and I know it's tough on them. My sister and I have always been real close. She was always very supportive and never held anything back. She asks the doctor for all the details.

Q. Can you explain in one word, or one sentence, your real gut feeling about the cis-platinum treatment?

A. The first day I went through cis-platinum was absolutely, without a doubt, the worst day of my whole life—THE WORST DAY OF MY LIFE—it was! I was so psyched up with OH COME ON, LET'S GO, LET'S DO IT. I was so high literally and mentally and I fell to earth in such a fast time it was the hardest crash of my life. What made it worse was that I had an adverse reaction to Reglan (drug injections to prevent the severe nausea). This stuff was surging through my body. It overpowered my body with so hot a sensation, a burning really. Really bad! It didn't keep me from getting sick. I kept going in and out of trances. The doctor came at 1:30 in the morning and ordered drugs to stop the reaction (I couldn't breathe). I was transferred to Jefferson Hospital right away. Cis-platinum chemo is something that is really, really hard to explain to anybody. It's a sick—a sick I don't think normally you can get that sick outside of the hospital. I've had cis-platinum five times now, and I can remember my inner feelings each time thinking, OH, THE HECK WITH IT—IT'S NOT WORTH IT—but you always gotta remember that it does end, so if you keep that in the back of your mind it helps. You're not real worried about what tomorrow will be like at the time—you feel if you could have just one minute's peace (from nausea and exhaustion), just give me even thirty seconds, just not this suffering for awhile, you'll settle for thirty seconds. I would say for seven days after cis-platinum my body is totally drained. I lose about 8 pounds every time I get it, but I gain the pounds back.

Q. Dave, can you watch the cis-platinum drip from the bag, or does that offend you?

A. The last time I got cis-platinum in the morning, and I sat there looking at the chemotherapy thinking, "This thing saves lives, but it also—it's a great, great thing, but a terrible, terrible thing at the same time. To get better you have to get so much worse and it is very, very hard to look at the cis-platinum dripping. You wouldn't want to do it unless you really have to; you wouldn't want to wish it on anybody...Anybody I ever hear of who is going through cis-platinum will have all my sympathy. It's a lot easier on yourself if you have a positive outlook.

Dave tolerates other chemotherapy treatments quite well, e.g., weekly shots of Velban. "I take it all okay except the cis-platinum," says Dave.

Q. Dave, were there some thoughts about the disease that you did not or could not share with others?

A. Yes, when you're in bed at night is when you get into praying. I did a lot—a lot—of praying. I always felt that...I said to HIM, "You're going to do with me whatever you're going to do with me, but you know that I really want to live and I'm fighting this the best I can." Looking up at the ceiling Dave said—"I hope YOU ARE IMPRESSED!!!"

But I wasn't afraid to go to bed at night. I was very comfortable with myself. It's when I am by myself and I can definitely think—that's when you do your best thinking. You're not going to go around thinking or saying there is a possibility that you could die, but I think that's something that's always in the back of your mind in the early going stages. It bothered me knowing that you could die, but if that's what was going to happen, I was going to do my darndest to live, but I was never afraid of dying. I was doing everything I could. It was cancer against me. But one of the main things is that the oncologist said I was going to get better, and that was my main belief. Anger was my first reaction hearing I had cancer, but that passed just as quickly as it came.

Q. Are you more appreciative of life now, Dave?

A. Oh, absolutely, sure. You realize life can be taken away from you.

Q. Were there some people you heard from that you hadn't expected to hear from when you became ill, Dave, or was there someone you expected to reach out to you and he did not?

A. I have one aunt—and this upset me, but I could understand. When we were talking a little while ago, she said even when she heard my name, it made her sick to her stomach because of the thought I had cancer. She's never called me in the hospital, and she's a very close aunt of mine, so some people can't deal with it.

Q. What do you think of the medical profession, mainly the handling of you during your illness? In particular, how do you feel about the doctor's treatment of you?

A. I think he is terrific. You said it before when you told me one patient you know considers him next to God.

Q. Do you feel he answers your questions for you?

A. He answers your questions to the point, short. It might not be the answer you want to hear but it's always an honest answer—just not always what you want to hear.

Q. Dave, what were your initial reactions to the other patients in the oncologist's office? What do you think of the atmosphere there?

A. You would never know these people have cancer; they're wide open, talking about everything, hardly ever talking about the disease. I was real surprised when I went there.

Q. Dave, was there anyone in particular who gave you a special boost, a shot in the arm, so to speak, about how you were handling your disease? You know, sometimes a person will make a statement to you that later strengthens you, perhaps such a statement as, "You make me comfortable because you are so able to handle your problems." Was there any such statement you can recall that made you realize you were also helping someone else through your illness?

A. I got a shot in the arm about the third time I was in for cis-platinum treatments. My cousin died, and his wife says I helped her by giving them inspiration. I was worried because she had helped me so much by giving me money to go to New York to have a lot of tests done. She took me to the American Oncologist Hospital for an interview. I was worried about them (his cousin and wife) and rightfully so, but that was a terrible feeling. I always pray that nothing happens to anybody I know or anyone in the family while I'm in the hospital, cause there's not a darn thing you can do except be by yourself to think.

Q. What about your future, Dave? What has changed about your plans, if anything, due to the fact you have had cancer? (Dave does not address the subject of health; instead he speaks of yet another ramification of a long term illness.)

A. I thought I'd be more financially independent than I am right now. It set me back awhile. But I have a good job now and everything is working its way up.

Q. Are there any positive aspects of your life that have resulted from being ill?

A. I think there's one outstanding one. It's funny how something like this pulls a family together, and it's terrible something like this has to happen to do it—to get everybody together in one room at a certain time, but I think it's definitely done that.

Q. And what are the negative results or feelings brought about by this, Dave?

A. Hospitals!!! Although the nurses are great, there is better individual care in suburban hospitals as versus large metropolitan hospitals. Although I'm amazed at the tests they can do at Jefferson Hospital. A lot of people will get cancer and it's better, if you're going to get it, to get it while you're young and while you can handle it better.

Dave became a bit pensive for a few moments...I watched and waited for him to offer verbally the thoughts that were obviously running through his mind. His eyes dimmed and saddened as he said, "Cancer is a terrible word. They ought to change the word."

"What would they change it to, Dave?" I asked.

"Oh, I don't know, but I think there are a lot of people being cured from it right now, but people don't hear of that. The only thing people think of is death with cancer. It's simultaneous with death. And I'll bet you it will be wiped out soon, I think so! I think if your body can handle the chemotherapy, you're probably halfway through."

We smiled at one another as the nurse entered the room to prepare him for the sixth and final cis-platinum treatment.

14.
Second Surgery

There is nothing to fear
but fear itself!

Franklin Roosevelt

October 14, 1981

.....Dawn peeks through my bedroom window searching for my leaf. Looking for signs of vibrancy. It has faded. I think I too have faded in and out of a light sleep on this autumn morning. The family sounds bustle around me. They clatter and slam their collective way into another day.

When I am alone I call the oncologist and confirm the date....November 2, 1981. That night I tell them. More surgery. I answer the questions they ask, and even some they do not, cannot ask.

I discard the leaf. Outside, the snap of autumn beckons. More leaves are swirling today. New ones. They too, as if by magic, prance and dance earth-bound and beautiful.

Surgery cannot be as difficult as the first day and night I spend here. I am on the cancer floor and the devastation of this disease presses upon me as I walk along this hall. There is a poignancy too piercing to ignore here.

After my first walk I resolve not to do this again. It is too close here. The sounds of the struggle crawling under closed doors and the signs of it there to see at every open doorway. Families sit with heads bowed. A sinister silence hovers high above the room as the loved one is watched. OH GOD, I hug my bed and steel myself against the fear that drifts in on me here; nightmarish and dark.

Despair is a heartbeat away and I look frantically for my Spiritual Trio and my positive attitude. Meditate...it escapes me now...in this day and throughout this night. The quiet screams at me. Dying sounds of patients, my brothers and sisters-in-arms losing the fight here.

They have been where I am and I am terrified at going to the place where they reside.

I stay in my bed and fight with myself. I grapple to keep my courage around me like a wet sheet in an ice storm. I pray for these fellow sufferers and wait for my hour and another nexus in my life. I am afraid and alone.

The nurses here were special. Compassionate and caring and, I think, understaffed. My surgeon and his staff work to keep me informed. They sat with me, generous with their time, and ran through all that would transpire later that day. I unveiled my fears to them and I felt confident now. My fears were: is my heart strong enough for this surgery; what will happen should I encounter breathing difficulties; am I going to die?

I fear the loss of control when unconscious. The psychiatrists can deal with that!

I will be on a breathing machine during surgery. As an added precaution my heart will be constantly monitored. The surgeon explains all possibilities:

1) I can get hepatitis

2) There is difficulty matching my bloodtype. I may need a transfusion during surgery. I learned that blood given me during cisplatinum treatments was not compatible.

3) I may have a resection of the bowel. I'll know immediately because a tube will be protruding from my mouth for drainage.

4) Nodes will be removed and sent for biopsy.

5) Growing tumors could be involved. Tumor he can excise he will.

6) Cancer cells that look like sand will be destroyed by radiation treatments after surgery.

This surgeon is frank and comprehensive and I am well prepared for tomorrow. I lie awake and consider all of this.

I am weary and ready at the same time. This is my moment and I have prepared for this for 21 months...

DARE I HOPE???!!!

I AM ALIVE. I am wheeled through bright hallways to my room. There are smiling faces. I AM ALIVE. This place is alive. The dread is gone. The fear is disappeared. I AM ALIVE!

Hands touch the blankets that cover me. I am wheeled past my family and they are all smiles. They caress me and their warmth comes through to me and dulls the pain and makes this world a wonderful place again.

"Honey, it's okay. You made it!" That was Bill. "The doctor is pleased, Mom. He's pleased." "I love you. You did great. Just fine!"

Their words reach through to me. I cannot cogently respond. "My trio did it again," I manage. My words are unrecognizable. My smile articulates everything.

That night my hand feels through the fog of the waning anesthesia. There is no tube in my mouth. My bandana covers my bald head. The surgical cap is gone.

At mid-morning the following day I get my report from the surgeon: the hysterectomy is complete, a tumor on the bowel is removed; they cut through the adhesions and biopsied the stomach; they removed small unidentified specks from the pelvis and took out the fat-pad lining the pelvic tissue; they took biopsies of both upper and lower abdomen. Now we wait for results. This takes five days.

Surely...I felt...surely...

A young doctor from the medical team burst into my room, nearly breathless. "DO I HAVE GOOD NEWS FOR YOU." She waved a piece of paper. "The biopsies are all back," she said. Sigmoid, rectosigmoid, cul-de-sac, periaoretic fat-pad, omentum...NO EVIDENCE OF TUMOR!

The uterus contained benign tumor of the smoothe muscle, ectopic endometriosis present. NO TUMOR! Right and left common iliac nodes reveal reactive hyperplasia with fatty infiltrates. NO TUMOR!

She reached down and enveloped me in her arms, tears of joy streaming down her face. I joined her.

My hospital door hung on hinges of joy. Throughout the day residents and members of the nursing staff popped in to congratulate me. A resident stood beside my bed. "It's so seldom we have this opportunity to share such good results." They really cared and felt free to express it and stay and share my joy for a few moments that day. I wept with joy and exhaustion.

The invisible barrier was down. These health professionals passed through it willingly to share this with me.

My clinical knowledge was limited and I did not totally understand the litany of names given to the various tissues tested. One phrase leaped up from the jargon and thrilled me: NO TUMOR. Perhaps that's all I really wanted to hear.

The oncologist stood at the foot of my bed. "No visible evidence of active cancer cells," he said. His pleasure was open. I'll never know if he would have come closer. I stunned him. "Has a patient ever said 'I love you'," I asked. He abruptly left the room mumbling his reply. (I'm sure he was blushing.)

Later that day I overheard my roommate and her husband. "You can't help but feel happy for her," he said. Her reply brought the larger reality of this place back into focus. "Oh, but I'm sure she's overreacting," she said. She was a cancer patient and her struggle for her life was very close to her.

Two days after my surgery I was seated in a chair, suddenly aware of laughter and swift movement in the hall. The sign caught me first: "HURRAY FOR MOM," scrawled on a silver helium-filled balloon. It was a balloon tree and it was mine.

The colors caught me—yellow, rust and green flowing from ribbons of gold and brown. Oddly they reminded me of my leaf, another gift from the autumn of 1981.

Conclusion

Leaving the hospital was odd. I was weary of the battle and wary of what my new life would bring. I was going to be well after all. Psychologically I had not yet adjusted I suppose. I thought how I would adjust with time; and thought again how very differently I now approached time.

I never asked God, "Why me" when I was diagnosed. I wanted to avoid that now too. I wanted to take it as it came to me and move on. Life was waiting and time was so very different now. I wanted to move forward.

I want to share two incidences with you as I close:

1) The oncologist later informs me it is advisable that I continue with weekly chemotherapy for an additional year and a half; just in case! I agree. I trust. We have come a long way.

2) On my first solo outing, January 1982, I went to a local gift store. "Gee, I haven't seen you in a long time Mrs. Quain," said the lady shop-keeper. "I heard you had cancer." "My brother has cancer, and he is very ill, has lost all his hair and is taking chemotherapy for six months. He is so weak from the treatments." Then, to my utter amazement and chagrin, she added, "Aren't you glad you had the easy kind?"!

Afterword

Directions for Visiting a Hospitalized Cancer Patient.

1) Just inside the door of the patient's room, mention the patient's name aloud, to make him/her aware of your presence. Pause briefly at the foot of the bed to see if patient is awake. If you are unsure that patient recognizes you, immediately tell him/her your name. A sick patient should not be challenged to identify a visitor. When you mention your own name it prevents this problem from occurring.

Ask patient if this is a good time to visit. If it is OK then begin visit. If it is not an ideal time patient may ask you to wait a few minutes until he/she is prepared for company. Patient may want to:

a) rinse his/her mouth

b) comb/brush hair

c) go to bathroom

d) change hospital gown he/she is wearing

e) need assistance from a nurse for some personal reason such as a change of soiled bed linens or removal of a bedpan.

2) Once patient has given OK, immediately pass beyond the foot of the patient's bed, along the bedside that patient is facing. This prevents ill person from having to change his/her position in bed. Be certain you physically pass beyond the foot of the patient's bed to converse with him/her. Failure to come within close proximity causes a variety of reactions for a

113

seriously ill person. Reluctance to get near the patient can be interpreted as:

a) Bad news is forthcoming from visitor.

b) Visitor is afraid of coming too close to patient for a variety of reasons. Such as:

—fear of an offensive odor.

—changes in the patient's physical appearance has frightened visitor.

—attached intravenous tubes, or draining apparatus are offensive to visitor.

—visitor may be afraid of 'catching' disease from patient.

3) Always make an effort to maintain direct eye contact with the patient. This gesture is both reassuring and convincing. It gives a patient trust in what is being said.

4) If you are comfortable with touching—touch the patient. A critically ill person is very vulnerable, in need of TLC. Hence a touch is similar to a pat on the back, a warming gesture. The visitor might want to simply touch bed clothing near side of patient's body. This will disturb bed clothes and generate a sense of touch (caring). Or perhaps an impersonal body part, covered by bed linens, might be touched. Such as: the ankle, calf or knee. If patient is receptive to touching it is more desirable to touch the patient's hand. All these touching suggestions are non-intimate contacts.

5) If the visitor can handle the gravity of the situation or if the visitor wants to allow the patient a willing ear to discuss the illness it is appropriate to lead the conversation in that direction. This verbal compassion can result in allowing the patient a release of his pent up emotions. Tears may be shed by both patient and visitor, and that is OK—it cleanses the heart. Fears may be addressed and that too is OK, as long as visitor can

handle the situation. A visitor must remember it is difficult to talk about and frightening to hear aspects of this disease. If the patient does not want to discuss these issues with the visitor he/she will say just that. No offense should be taken.

6) A seriously ill patient will generally respond well to the following statements:

a) "The news you heard must be upsetting!"

b) "It hurts me knowing you are ill (or suffering)"

c) "This must be a painful experience for you." Emotional, mental, and physical pain may be talked about.

d) "Did the doctor see you *today?*"

e) "Did he give you any *new* information?"

f) "How are you feeling *now?*"

The words *today, new* and *now* bring the conversation to the present time. The present time is what the patient wants to talk about. He isn't making long range plans. And is often absorbed in the present.

7) To help a patient cope it is important that someone associated with the patient try to ascertain if the patient is under any other stress, other than the gigantic stress of a life threatening diagnosis. Many patients are more concerned about their families, or family situations, than they are about their own physical condition.

8) Less serious but equally important conversations can be started by the visitor asking the patient about his/her past activities. Work, school, hobbies, politics, current events, history in the making, etc. It is important to bring the news of the outside world to an alert patient.

9) In all visits to a hospitalized patient it is of utmost importance to be aware of patient's energy level. Do not tire the patient by staying for a lengthy amount of time. Being attuned to the patient's body language will enable one to understand if patient is too tired, unreceptive, or uncomfortable. The first priority is the patient's well being.

10) Do not UNDER ANY CIRCUMSTANCE visit a cancer patient, in treatment or following surgery, if you the visitor are ill. Be aware the patient's immune system is weakened and you do not want to jeopardize his/her health any further than already exist.

The above suggestions apply not only to visitors but in many instances to medical professionals as well.

11) For physicians, nurses: A patient is reinforced by clear, concise and informative discussion with those in whom he is developing trust. Most patients respect the truth. The greatest fears develop because IMAGINING IS WORSE THAN KNOWING.

And Should the Outcome Be Otherwise

What appropriate words can a person offer to the survivors of a deceased cancer patient. A very difficult situation often leaves us speechless. Yet most people want to offer some appropriate words of comfort, either verbal or written expressions of sympathy. The following phrases have been well received by the bereaved:

a) "How sad I am to hear of the death of your (wife, husband, mother, father, son, daughter, grandparent, friend, etc.).

b) No greater gift could (name of deceased) have than being loved by (name of survivor(s)).

c) No greater gift would (name of deceased) want than to be loved by so many.

d) Please take comfort in knowing (name of deceased) would have chosen not to suffer anymore.

e) Living to the point of intolerable pain and watching those who love us suffer an intolerable grief is the last mile one cares to walk. Our comfort now is knowing his/her pain is over.

f) My prayers are with you, my love I give you.

g) What we will do now is treasure our memories of (name of deceased).